T0329694

The Oocyte Economy

The
Oocyte
Economy

The Changing Meaning of Human Eggs

....

Catherine Waldby

DUKE UNIVERSITY PRESS · DURHAM AND LONDON · 2019

© 2019 Duke University Press
All rights reserved
Printed and bound by CPI Group (UK) Ltd, Croydon, CR0 4YY

Designed by Matthew Tauch
Typeset in Scala Pro and Helvetica Neue
by Westchester Publishing Services

Library of Congress Cataloging-in-Publication Data
Names: Waldby, Catherine, [date] author.
Title: The oocyte economy : the changing meaning
of human eggs / Catherine Waldby.
Description: Durham : Duke University Press, 2019. |
Includes bibliographical references and index.
Identifiers: LCCN 2018047204 (print)
LCCN 2018059627 (ebook)
ISBN 9781478005568 (ebook)
ISBN 9781478004110 (hardcover : alk. paper)
ISBN 9781478004721 (pbk. : alk. paper)
Subjects: LCSH: Ovum. | Fertility, Human—Social
aspects. | Fertility, Human—Economic aspects. |
Human reproductive technology—Economic aspects. |
Infertility—Treatment—Economic aspects. |
Medical tourism.
Classification: LCC RG133.5 (ebook) | LCC RG133.5 .W35 2019
(print) | DDC 618.1/7806—dc23
LC record available at https://lccn.loc.gov/2018047204

Contents

....

Acknowledgments

....

The research for this study was supported by two Australian Research Council (ARC) grants: "The Oöcyte Economy: The Changing Meanings of Human Eggs in Fertility, Assisted Reproduction and Stem Cell Research" ARC Professorial Future Fellowship, and "Human Oöcytes for Stem Cell Research: Donation and Regulation in Australia" Linkage Project, with CIS Ian Kerridge and Loane Skene, postdoctoral fellow Katherine Carroll, and doctoral student Margaret Boulos. I was also given access to some of the primary interview data from the research program "Regenerative Medicine in Europe: Emerging Needs and Challenges in a Global Context" EU FP7 project. My thanks to Andrew Webster, Kathrin Braun, and Suzanne Schultz for their generosity in this regard.

Earlier versions of the material in chapter 7 have appeared in *Culture, Health and Sexuality* (Waldby 2015a), the *Journal of Cultural Economy* (Waldby 2015b), and *Social Science and Medicine* (Waldby et al. 2013). An earlier version of some of the material in chapter 3 has appeared in *Sociology of Health and Illness* (Waldby and Carroll 2012). In the cases of the two coauthored papers, I have returned to the original datasets, carried out my own reanalysis of the interview and focus group material, and substantially amended, updated, and recontextualized the argument and analysis.

As with any book-length project, I have incurred many debts and have many colleagues, friends, and family to thank. First, I am grateful to all the women interviewed over a period of ten years, in Australia, the UK, and the United States, whose candor and generosity have made this study possible. In the same vein, I wish to thank the CEOs, clinicians, embryologists, stem cell scientists, counseling staff, ethicists, and other professionals whom I either interviewed or consulted during the study, and who provided generous access to their programs.

Expert research assistance and invaluable insight was provided at various times by Rachel Carr, Michelle Jamieson, Brydan Leanne, Kim McLeod, and Susannah French.

My thanks to my generous colleagues and interlocutors: Stine Adrian; Rene Almeling; Kathrin Braun; Katherine Carroll, there from the beginning; Adele Clarke and the terrific grad students at UCSF; Haidan Chen; the indispensable Melinda Cooper; Sheryl Delacey; Donna Dickenson; Maria Fanin; the late Herbert Gottweis, much missed; Christian Haddad; Erica Haimes; Johanna Hood; Klaus Lindgaard Høyer; Isabel Karpin; Helen Keane; Ian Kerridge; Charlotte Kroløkke; Thomas Lemke; Nina Lykke; Ann McGrath; Catherine Mills; Dean Murphy; Michel Nahman; Bronwyn Parry, Anne Pollock, Barbara Prainsack and Nikolas Rose at Kings College, London, for always welcoming me when I'm in town; Kaushik Sunder Rajan; Celia Roberts; Jackie Leach Scully; Loane Skene; Cameron Stuart; Karen Throsby; Ayo Wahlberg; Andrew Webster; Andrea Whittaker; Sonja Van Wichelen; and Clare Williams. My apologies to anyone I have forgotten. My gratitude also goes to the Research School of Social Sciences at ANU, for providing such a stellar environment, and to Rae Frances, Paul Pickering, and Vice Chancellor Brian Schmidt for inspiration and support.

As always a special thank you to my friends, interlocutors, and colleagues Warwick Anderson, Susan Kippax, and Pamela Hansford, for too many forms of support and intelligent exchange to feasibly list; to my partner, Paul Jones, for the care, love, intellectual generosity, and forbearance that allowed me to both start and complete this project while remaining comparatively sane; and to my family, David, Valerie, Maddison, Sebastian, and Gavan Waldby, as well as Jenny Hill, for their love and support.

Introduction

....

This book addresses a particular cell lineage—human oocytes, the gametes or reproductive cells specific to women. These are the cells that transmit genetic inheritance from mother to child and orchestrate the processes of conception and gestation. At the broadest level, in this book, I ask what it means to live with this cell lineage. How does its particular history, trajectory, and affordances intersect with the biological and social lives of women? How do women experience and understand the capacities and constraints of these cells, and how do they incorporate them into their everyday lives as an element of reproductive practice?

These are questions nicely located at the pivot point between nature and culture. As biological questions, they interrogate the relationship between part and whole, cellular life and organism life. Our bodies, like those of all complex organisms, are constituted of cell matrices that cooperate in our coherence. Each kind has its own evolutionary history. Our bodies are ecosystems that assemble cellular communities, which lead back into evolutionary time (Dupré 2012). The exquisite coordination of lymphocytes, macrophages, and B cells that orchestrates our immune system and defeats viral and bacterial infection plays out ancient dynamics among the earliest microbial life. The capacity of our gut to digest food depends on the vast array of symbiotic bacteria that have coevolved with more complex organisms like ourselves and that lend us functional capacities to metabolize what we eat (Ley et al. 2008). Our blood, with its complex components—hemoglobin, erythrocytes, leukocytes, plasma— and its salinity identical to sea water, recapitulates an evolutionary history that leads back to invertebrate life in the primitive oceans (Cooper 1976). Our cells cooperate in our organism life. Basal nuclei are subsumed into the larger structures of the brain, so that they serve the entire body rather than local stimuli (Sarnat and Netsky 2002). Cardiomyocytes bundle into cardiac muscle, so that their contractile force create a heartbeat (Gutstein et al. 2003). The qualities of organism life that emerge from this cooperation are nevertheless contingent and indebted to the material specificities of the cells themselves. Cardiomyocytes may lose their communicative capacities and become arrhythmic, out of sync, so that the heart no longer provides stable support for blood circulation (Harvey and Leinwand 2011). All our cells may immortalize themselves, losing their ability to die. Immortalized cells form tumors, disrupting other organs and the very life of the afflicted. The life of the cell and the life of the organism coincide imperfectly, and their cooperation is partial. In the case of oocytes, their fertile capacity is not simply at the service of the women who embody them. Many women find that their projects and plans are at odds with this capacity, and their experience of this disjuncture forms one of the major themes of this study.

As cultural questions, they interrogate the historical nature of embodiment. Fertility as a human capacity is ordered and highly meaningful for all cultures, dependent as they are for their continuity on the ability of their members to bear children. My question can be considered properly, however, only for quite particular social locations and historical moments. Prior to the middle of the twentieth century, oocytes as a tissue simply formed part of the in vivo texture of fertile experience, rather than as a distinct element. Since the mid-twentieth century, biologists, clinicians, and women themselves have sought technical traction on human oocytes, as a means of controlling fertility more generally. A protracted history of experimentation, first in invertebrates and nonhuman mammals, then in humans, created the conditions for clinical in vitro fertilization (IVF) in the late 1970s. The protocols for IVF isolated and externalized oocytes so that they could be manipulated through laboratory procedures. This opened the way for an ever-expanding suite of technical services that give women with the necessary income the ability to manipulate and order their oocytes and try to bring them into line with their life course.

Such services are attractive because oocytes as a cell lineage involve a particular set of temporal constraints. Their biology is characteristically parsimonious and atretic. The rarest of cells in the human body, they mature one by one, each lunar month, and most women produce only four hundred mature oocytes over their lifetimes. Women lose their fertile capacity steadily in the first half of a typical lifetime, so that few conceive after the age of forty. This biological schedule is more and more at odds with the costs of household formation and the demands of credentialing and professionalization that characterize the life course of middle-class women in postindustrial democracies. As more and more women seek higher education, demanding careers, and the satisfactions of the public world, they also find that they must grapple with the intransigence of their oocyte biology, if they wish to have children.[1] Techniques that defer oocyte fertility, compensate for their intrinsic parsimony, or access those of another woman are highly valued by women who discover that they may not be ready to conceive in their twenties or early thirties. The demand for IVF and other assisted reproductive technologies (ARTs) has accelerated year on year in Australia, the UK, and the United States throughout the early twenty-first century, driven primarily by women in their mid- to late thirties or early forties (Human Fertilisation and Embryology Authority 2016; Macaldowie, Lee, and Chambers 2015; Centers for Disease Control and Prevention 2017). Beyond the Anglosphere, reproductive epidemiologists estimate that global use of assisted reproduction is increasing by 9 percent per year, and they report that women over forty make up a steadily increasing proportion of fertility patients (Dyer et al. 2016).

This book is largely concerned with the social relations that inform and are elaborated around this body of technique. In this sense, it is not an anthropological investigation into the human meanings of fertility, but rather a more specific "tissue economy" account. Since my work on the Visible Human Project, in the late 1990s, I have investigated human tissue economies across several different tissue types—cadaveric (Waldby 2000), blood and solid organs (Waldby and Mitchell 2006), embryonic and hematopoetic stem cells (Waldby 2006; Gottweis, Salter, and Waldby

2009), oocyte donation (Carroll and Waldby 2012; Boulos, Kerridge, and Waldby 2014), and multiple studies, with Melinda Cooper, that focus on the relationship between women's reproductive biological materials and biological innovation in therapuetic cloning and stem cell treatments (Waldby and Cooper 2008, 2010; Cooper and Waldby 2014).

This study builds on this body of scholarship in that it shares a concern with how forms of circulation and valuation made possible by biomedical technique condition the significance of the tissue. The idea of a tissue economy is that donated human tissues (blood, embryos, organs, sperm, oocytes) have a productivity that can be ordered in different ways. While still inside the donor's body, tissues are part of the self and help to sustain the person. Once donated, they can sustain the life and health of the recipients (as in blood and organ donation); they may be banked for future use (for example, cord blood); or they may become elements in laboratory research (for example, embryonic stem cell lines). In each case, tissues are procured, managed, banked, and circulated in a system designed to maximize their latent productivity. Within the body, different tissues have different qualities and capacities—blood oxygenates the organs, while bone marrow generates the blood system itself, for example. Once donated, these qualities necessarily delimit the kinds of circulation possible for the tissue. Its capacity as transferable material is shaped at the intersection of its function in the body, its durability, its immunological specificity, and the kinds of technical and social systems available to procure, potentiate, store, and distribute it.

Reproductive tissues introduce an additional complexity here, because they form intermediate materials between two different bodies, the parental and the offspring. The tissues may constitute and sustain prenatal life—the gametes in conception, and the placental, uterine, and cervical conditions that facilitate fetal existence—or they may sustain postnatal life, as breast milk is generated and provided to the infant. Oocytes play a pivotal role in the moment of conception, as do sperm, but they also lend themselves to the orchestration of the embryo and the gestational conditions of the pregnancy in a fashion that makes them particularly vital intermediary tissues in the processes of reproduction. This capacity is the quality that confers their value and forms the key to the oocyte economy.

Some tissues offer little affordance to technical intervention. The heart, kidneys, and most other solid organs are simply transferred between donor and recipient intact, with limited technical intervention in the

organ itself, although both donor and recipient bodies require prepara-
tion to facilitate the process. Blood was donated whole during the early
and mid-twentieth century but today is usually transferred in factions, as
plasma, for example, or as platelets that target specific conditions more
precisely than does whole blood. Some tissues are extremely time critical;
solid organs generally must be transferred between donor and recipient
within a few hours, involving complex cold-chain logistics and specialized courier services to avoid deterioration of the organ. Some tissues,
like cord blood, are readily frozen, while whole blood is not. The ability to
cryopreserve, to freeze and thaw, tissues is perhaps the single most important technique in the repertoire that shapes a tissue economy. Until very
recently, oocytes could only be donated fresh, a situation that has placed
striking constraints on their forms of circulation. One of the major themes
of this book is how a new capacity for cryopreservation is reshaping the
oocyte economy, from the most intimate transactions between a donor
and a recipient to the development of a global corporate market. Here we
will see how new technical developments can render formally intractable
tissues into more flexible, valuable substances.

A second feature of tissue economies is that they are not socially neutral but are *implicated in power relationships*. When a person donates tissue,
they make a bodily sacrifice in favor of another person, or of a research
program. Hence, the biotechnical capacity to transfer tissues immediately
raises questions of just distribution. Who should give tissues, under what
circumstances, and to whom? Oocytes are particularly mobile, dense points
at which such power relationships play out. While solid organ donation
(hearts, kidneys, livers, lungs) is managed in most jurisdictions according to principles of social equity, medical need, and humanitarian justice
(Healy 2006; Waldby and Mitchell 2006), oocytes are transacted under
more variable regulatory conditions. In some jurisdictions, such as the
Australian states and most northern European countries, oocytes are
treated according to the gift systems that order organ donation more
generally. They must be given altruistically and without inducement. No
jurisdiction, however, has succeeded in establishing a public gift system
for oocytes along the lines of national blood donation programs. Only a
tiny number of women will donate oocytes to strangers altruistically, so
women seeking such donors will generally wait in vain. In many other
places, however, oocyte provision is transactional. Young women sell
their oocytes to older women in exchange for money, although this is

habitually framed as compensation rather than frank payment (Cooper and Waldby 2014). This monetization is a quite exceptional feature of oocyte circulation. No other human tissue is so systematically ordered through significant money transactions, and this feature conditions the power relations between provider and recipient in particular ways.

In my research I have tackled this transactional aspect of the oocyte economy from two different directions. In my book with Melinda Cooper *Clinical Labor* (Cooper and Waldby 2014), we considered this economy from the point of view of production and labor, that is, with a focus on the *fertility providers*. We located oocyte transactions as one of the forms of embodied, transactional work associated with the lower echelons of the biomedical and pharmaceutical industries. We argued that oocyte provision should be understood as a specific kind of post-Fordist service work, continuous with but also distinct from the various forms of embodied service labor that proliferate in today's postindustrial economies. While this form of reproductive labor is typically framed as altruistic, and payment is framed as compensation, we set out the terms through which oocyte provision could be understood as a kind of fertility outsourcing. As in other forms of labor outsourcing, the oocyte vendor is constituted as an individual contractor who supplies the elements of fertility from outside the family proper in exchange for a fee.

In this book, I consider oocyte transactions from the other side of the relationship, as a practice of consumption and a kind of experience, as well as a form of economic relationship between different classes of women. I draw on 130 interviews with fertility clinicians and stem cell scientists, and women who have experience with fertility treatment, egg donation, egg freezing, and fertility tourism in Australia, the UK, and the United States. While some of the interviews were conducted with potential and actual oocyte *donors* in Australia, where donation is strictly regulated and noncommercial, the rest of the interviews were focused on the *acquisition* of oocytes, through international travel, and on the management of personal fertility through oocyte banking. In this sense the book is focused on a relatively privileged group—primarily middle-class, white, heterosexual, professional women living in the metropolitan centers of the Anglosphere. The cities of Sydney, London, and San Francisco feature here, cities with wealthy citizens and highly specialized service economies, where professional women can purchase niche forms of private clinical assistance to help them manage the refractory aspects of their fertile lives. The lives of oocyte vendors are in some cases quite similar—particularly in California, where vendors are typically highly credentialed, newly graduated women in their twenties—but in the majority of cases, oocyte vendors are drawn from the ranks of the precariat, women who work as undocumented cleaners and nannies in Spain, or young women from the former Eastern Bloc countries who travel to Greece and Cyprus to sell their eggs. The conditions of oocyte vending are examined at length in *Clinical Labor* (Cooper and Waldby 2014).

While this book focuses on the more privileged, consumption side of the oocyte economy, I do not want to imply that the experience portrayed here is less significant than that of the providers. Rather, the oocyte economy gives us a way to consider the deeply felt, affectively charged question of what fertility means to women who are still among the earliest generations for whom childbearing is largely elective. It also informs us about the conflicts across the life course of working women between the constraints of biology and the demands of credentialing and career establishment. The pattern of demographic and economic growth in advanced economies is increasingly determined by the fertility decisions of older women, who delay childbearing primarily because of concerns over affordability and the demands of working life (Commonwealth of Australia 2008). This cohort of women, however, is now faced with the growing body of medical evidence concerning age-related decline in the fertility of oocytes (Trounson and Godsen 2003). They turn in growing numbers to in vitro fertilization (IVF) and other kinds of assisted reproductive technology (ART) and hence must encounter the capacities and material constraints of their oocytes as a consequence of treatment.

Oocytes give particular insights into this situation precisely because they can be externalized, circulated, banked, transacted, and donated. Unlike most biological elements of female fertility—uterine, fallopian, cervical, which remain securely in vivo—oocytes have developed an ex vivo social life, and their significance for women mutates through these varied social locations. Like all human tissues, oocytes are charged with highly personal qualities. Their material constitution is marked by genetic, histological, and ontological qualities that link them irreducibly to their donors (Anderson 2008). Oocytes, as gametes, transmit the germ line, to use August Weismann's nineteenth-century term, "the living *hereditary substance*, which in all multicellular organisms, unlike the substance composing the perishable body of the individual, is transmitted from generation to generation" (Weismann 1892, xi). In Weismann's formulation, the gametes are the body's immortal cells, which transmit species being and family ancestry from generation to generation, while all other cells are somatic. Somatic cells constitute the body of the organism, but they are repeatedly replaced in its lifetime, and they are destined to die. In this sense oocytes transmit distinct historical qualities. They are profoundly associated with what I term in the book "generational time," the ways in which each woman locates herself in a family ancestry and a potential line of descent. Oocytes are the material capacities necessary to communicate generational time; they link the past and the future of the family through the woman's body. For women who feel the past and the future in this way, the ordering of their oocytes gives them a technical means to reconcile the demands of the present, particularly the demands of public life and individual performance, with this *longue durée* sense of inherited self, ancestral time, and obligation to continue the next generation.

For these reasons, oocytes have a particularly acute kind of value, associated with both their signal capacities to create and continue family and their rarity, their precipitous loss of capacity in the middle of the life course. This personal value has been complicated by their centrality in the business model of the private fertility sector, and more recently in the biomedical innovations associated with embryonic stem cell research and therapeutic cloning (Franklin 2013). This brings us to a third characteristic of tissue economies: *they are increasingly caught up in various kinds of capitalization and market value.* The life sciences are increasingly industrialized and configured as a bioeconomy, a form of wealth creation and commercial innovation that builds on the laboratory manipulation of vitality (OECD 2006; White House 2012).

The commercialization of oocytes dates from the early IVF era. During the 1980s, the new fertility treatments were largely classified as elective procedures by the National Health Service (NHS) in the UK (Lord et al. 2001) and as too difficult to regulate amid antiabortion politics in the United States (Jasanoff 2005). In Australia, since the early 1990s, a copayment system under Medicare has publicly subsidized IVF treatment, although there are routinely large gaps between fees set by the clinic and subsidy payments (Chambers, Hoang, and Illingworth 2013). In each case, fertility treatments were largely undertaken in private clinics as fee-for-service medicine. The production and management of patients' oocytes are essential elements of IVF treatment, and these technical skills are central to the sector's service provision and revenue generation. In many jurisdictions, brokerage, the procurement and curation of oocytes from desirable donors, creates an additional revenue stream for fertility clinics.

Oocytes also underpin some research sectors of the bioeconomy. Since the birth of Dolly the sheep in 1996, laboratories have sought human oocytes to try to replicate in humans the technique used to create Dolly, somatic cell nuclear transfer (SCNT). Although SCNT cannot be legally used for human reproduction, the method can be applied for *therapeutic* cloning, the creation of patient-specific stem cell lines. This demand for research oocytes has proved almost impossible to meet, however, as highly experimental laboratory requirements compete with reproductive demand. As I discuss in chapter 7 of this book, a handful of laboratories interested in SCNT have negotiated a workable procurement system through the professionalization of their providers and their inclusion within the value chain of innovation.

In this book, I aim to elucidate the consumption and innovation dynamics that inform the oocyte economy, but also the kinds of desire, imagination, and identity that animate it. The women interviewed for this study describe complex feelings about their oocytes, and they use them to reason, plan, and fantasize about both their past and their future. As tissues, oocytes are eminently relational, linking women back into their family history, laterally into their relationships with husbands and partners, and forward into their relationships with children, actual or potential. Women unable to produce sufficient oocytes to conceive through IVF describe a sense of bereavement, the erasure of a relational capacity that they had assumed was theirs. Donated or purchased oocytes link provider to recipient, often in terms that the women interviewed found difficult to reconcile. The oocyte economy, in other words, accounts for systems of value locatable in both public and private worlds, in commerce and in family, at global and intimate scales.

Fieldwork and Data

The fieldwork for this book, supported by three grants, extends over three continents and eight years. The initial study, funded by the Australian Research Council (ARC) and carried out between 2008 and 2011, involved a research collaboration with a Sydney fertility clinic, investigating women's preparedness to donate oocytes for research.[2] Three participant groups were interviewed: twenty women who were ex-IVF patients, five reproductive oocytes donors, and six clinical and counseling staff. Focus groups were organized with fourteen young women (aged thirty and under), with no direct experience of IVF, regarding their understandings of and feelings about donating oocytes for research. As the field methods were face to face and qualitative, we also gathered extensive contextual knowledge about how women understand and value their oocytes, how they felt about giving them, and under what circumstances they might consider such a gift (Carroll and Waldby 2012; Waldby and Carroll 2012; Waldby et al. 2012, 2013; Boulos 2014; Boulos, Kerridge, and Waldby 2014).

The second study, carried out from 2008 to 2010, investigated the understandings of stem cell scientists and regulators about oocyte donation for research, funded as part of the European Union's Regenerative Medicine in Europe FP7 project. The chief investigators, Kathrin Braun and Susanne Schultz, interviewed forty-five key informants in Europe and in California (Braun and Schultz 2012), and they generously gave me access to their transcripts for this book. As my focus is on Australia, the UK, and California, however, I have made use of only the fourteen interviews that correspond to those locations.

The third study, supported by my ARC Future Fellowship, focused on cross-border oocyte transactions and the implications of new vitrification technologies for women and the fertility industry.[3] This involved interviews with thirty-three clinical, laboratory, and business staff in Sydney, Brisbane, London, San Francisco, and Phoenix, Arizona. I also interviewed fifteen women who had banked their oocytes in London, and nine women based in Australia or the UK who had traveled overseas to obtain oocytes from a commercial donor. These interviews took place between 2012 and 2014. I pursued three additional interviews in the UK with clinicians and ethicists involved in mitochondrial donation during 2015. In each of the chapters that deals with this material, I provide more detail about the interviews. The appendix lists all the nonprofessional interviewees by pseudonyms and gives some information about their circumstances, while professional interviewees are described by their position in the main text only. The Human Research Ethics Committee of the University of Sydney granted ethical approval for this research.

Hence the data presented here give snapshots of particular questions in particular locations at particular times with particular kinds of informants.[4] The time line these data describe maps some of the key developments in both stem cell research and fertility medicine, particularly the global regulatory fallout from the Hwang scandal in 2005 (see chapter 7), the dwindling of scnt funding after the development of induced pluripotent stem cells in 2006, and the repercussions of oocyte vitrification and the growth of medical tourism on these sectors.[5] The time line also tracks how the notions of a "fertility cliff" and a "biological clock" have become key reference points in women's popular culture, in marked distinction to the celebration of late motherhood in women's media during the 1990s (Jermyn 2008).

The three salient urban locations—Sydney, London, and San Francisco—provide some degree of comparability in demographics: each of them is a global city with a high-cost, high-service economy, a center of innovation and finance, with the kind of relatively wealthy professional population of women who typically form the client base for fertility treatments. At the same time, each location provides important kinds of comparisons around regulation. Australia has maintained a conservative, anticommercial ethos regarding oocyte donation. The UK has taken a more liberal approach to procurement since the advent of egg sharing in the late 1990s, and since 2009, it has moved toward payment of significant compensation (£750, or US$1,000, at time of writing), which attracts providers while staying within the terms of European Union (EU) anticommercialization laws around tissue donation (Human Fertilisation and Embryology Authority 2015a). California has anticommercial statutes, but in practice, oocyte providers are paid for fertility services, and the state has an extremely vigorous clinical and brokerage sector dedicated to the curation of desirable oocyte genetics. These regulatory differences produce quite different systems of oocyte procurement and management, as well as niche services to circumvent them.

These particularities illuminate some dimensions of the oocyte economy and fail to account for others. When possible, I have drawn on secondary data, particularly from the excellent feminist research on arts more generally and extensive historical and regulatory research to enrich the primary data at my disposal. I do not claim to give a comprehensive account but rather draw on the breadth of approaches to consider what oocytes mean and how they are valued, for women, for the clinicians and embryologists who work with them, and for the research scientists who hope to leverage their reanimating powers in various ways.

Experience and Method

While the research presented here draws extensively on expert informants and biomedical research, it also engages directly with the more experiential, affective, and embodied dimensions of the oocyte economy. The majority of research for this book involved face-to-face, one-to-one interviews, over one to two hours. In most cases, these interviews proceeded at the participant's home, sometimes with children and partner present, sometimes not. In every case, the interviews involved discussion of experiences considered private, highly personal, and distinctly emotional. They touched on the desire for children, the difficult negotiations with partners, the onerous and often distressing nature of fertility treatment, the failed cycles, the miscarriages, the hope invested in frozen eggs or embryos, and the woman's sense of her life course and how it mediated relationships between different generations and family histories. In some cases, particularly in the interviews with women who had frozen their eggs, the discussion touched on painful relationship breakups, divorce, and the bleakness of life contemplated without a partner and children.

In the interviews I conducted, participants were often angry, frustrated, or grief stricken, regretful, and sometimes tearful. My colleague Katherine Carroll, who also conducted a portion of the interviews, notes the highly personal, sometimes distressing emotional tenor:

> Asking about the IVF experience and the willingness of women undergoing IVF to donate embryos or eggs involves hearing about the most intimate of concerns: tales of repeated failed attempts at pregnancy without IVF, then repeated failed IVF treatments, miscarriages, emotional distress, financial hardship and in some cases, even domestic violence, eviction and incarceration. The interview may also touch on career achievements and failed marriages, often at the cost of starting a family in fertile years. These stories are shared over a cup of tea, a glass of juice, while holding the baby, meeting the husband or engaging with the toddler. (Carroll 2013, 552)[6]

Carroll explicitly engages with this emotional tenor to argue that qualitative, face-to-face research about fertility and reproductive experience, like many other domains of feminist research, requires a particularly intense kind of emotional labor from the interviewer. On the one hand, the interview demands a receptive empathy, a nonjudgmental, open acceptance of the affective ethos the woman brings to her account, and on the other, it requires sufficient detachment to maintain the safety and ethical integrity of the interaction and the data it produces. The interview makes full sense only through a degree of identification between interviewer and participant, a sense of shared experience:

> Emotions and emotionality have traditionally been kept at bay in social research for reasons such as the fear of contaminating data, the difficulty of translating emotion into textual accounts or because of the fear emotional disclosure may have on professional academic careers. Thus, emotional and rational ways of knowing were placed in opposition, with the former occupying a lesser standing. However, it is clear that embodied, experiential and emotional ways of knowing pre-empt, coexist with and inform what is labelled "objective" knowledge. (Carroll 2013, 556)

This kind of empathic intersubjectivity can also be regarded as an entry point into broader social processes. While this study gives extensive attention to the experiential dimensions of the oocyte economy, I do not treat this experience as *self-evidently* significant. Rather, following Joan Scott's now canonical argument about the status of experience in history, I ask how experience counts as *evidence*, as data demanding social analytics and historiography. While experiential accounts are expressive of social relations, they cannot give such relations an exhaustive investigation, as Scott explains:

> How can we historicize "experience"? How can we write about identity without essentializing it? Answers to the second question ought to point toward answers to the first, since identity is tied to notions of experience, and since both identity and experience are categories usually taken for granted in ways that I am suggesting they ought not to be. It ought to be possible for historians to . . . make visible the assignment of subject-positions, not in the sense of capturing the reality of the objects seen, but of trying to understand the operations of the complex and changing discursive processes by which identities are ascribed, resisted, or embraced and which processes themselves are unremarked, indeed achieve their effect because they aren't noticed. (Scott 1992, 33)

Scott suggests that the particularity of experience can be read to open out the relationships between expressive self-formation, the self as felt and interiorized, and forms of subjectivity, the historically constituted, normative forms of social action available to particular selves. To interpret experience in this way involves identification of how the texture of every-day life and immersive time, the particularity of individual histories, are informed by the detail of social history. In this book, the women who offered their experience are knowingly or inadvertently informative about larger social dynamics—demography, gender, class, race, sexuality, kinship, biomedicine—and provide extremely rich accounts of what it means to live these dynamics as styles of life. A salient dimension of this experience derives from their close encounters with biomedicine as both a biological and a social force.

Michel Foucault's propositions about experience and history are help-ful here. Thomas Lemke notes the salience of experience as method in Foucault's later work, an articulation point that modulates the relation-ship between "forms of knowledge, mechanisms of power and relations to the self. It is this . . . tripartite 'matrix of experience' that reorients Fou-cault's work in the 1980s. Foucault gives up the original plan to study the history of sexuality . . . as 'a history of the experience of sexuality, where experience is understood as the correlation between fields of knowledge, types of normativity, and forms of subjectivity in a particular culture'" (Lemke 2011, 29).[7] This tripartite matrix is proposed at a high level of gener-ality. It becomes useful for the task at hand, however, because it suggests formative relations between scientific knowledge and the emergence of particular kinds of experience and identity. In Foucault's work, this for-mative relationship is most thoroughly explored in relation to the figure of the homosexual, a category as indebted for its coherence to nineteenth- and twentieth-century biomedicine as to actual sexual practice (Foucault 1978). In this study, I consider the ways in which the experience of wom-anhood in particular locations is inflected through the knowledge systems of fertility medicine and its capacity to administer women's reproductive biology. The ability to stimulate ovarian follicles, to retrieve multiple oo-cytes, and to fertilize, bank, or transfer them to another gives women's bodies and lives particular trajectories and constitutes particular webs of relationships. These relationships extend from the most proximate and intimate—those with a sexual partner and with a child—to kinship rela-tions both synchronic and diachronic, and from potential relationships with future loved ones to remote relations with oocyte providers, known and anonymized, in distant places.

To put it another way, the historical, normative associations connecting womanhood, femininity, and reproduction, the conditions of motherhood, are being rapidly reconstituted by clinical and commercial systems for the redistribution of reproductive capacity (Thompson 2005; Murphy 2012). The women interviewed for this study give poignant witness to both the possibilities and the constraints presented by this dynamic, as they relate their investigations, attempts, successes, and abrupt reversals in the bid for a child and a family. To this extent they also reanimate one of the lost etymologies of the term "experience": its relationship to "experiment."[8] In *Keywords*, Raymond Williams explores the shared terrain of these terms:

> Experience, in one main sense, was until the 18th Century, interchangeable with experiment (cf. modern French) from the common *experiri* [Latin]—to try, to put to the test. Experience . . . became not only a conscious test or trial but a consciousness of what has been tested or tried, and thence a consciousness of an effect or state. From [the sixteenth century] it took on a more general meaning, with more deliberate inclusion of the past (the tried and tested), to indicate knowledge derived from real events as well as from particular observation. Experiment, a noun of action, maintained the simple sense of a test or trial. (Williams 1983, 117)

This sense of experience, with its lineages in empirical experimentation and the history of science, lends itself particularly to the matter at hand. Women have entered courageously into highly experimental relationships with new reproductive technologies. Any advances made in this domain of medicine depend on this willingness to risk sometimes dangerous procedures and highly uncertain outcomes. This preparedness to risk oneself has historically been regarded by feminist commentators as evidence of a kind of false consciousness, of a lack of regard for oneself in the absence of a child, which demonstrates the internalization of patriarchal ideology. In chapter 2, dealing with the history of IVF, I try to reframe this willingness as part of a broader dynamic that encompasses the spectrum of reproductive self-experimentation, from the contraceptive activism of the early twentieth century to the newly chic social egg freezing of today.

In doing so, I try to give just and empathic witness to the experiences that form the substance of this book, and to fully consider the evidence they provide of the contemporary oocyte economy and of reproductive relationships more broadly. Rather than measuring these experiences against a particular set of articulated normative positions, I attempt to discern the ethos, quality of social experience, and lived meaning that the women interviewed felt for their oocytes. The practices of superovulation, of seeking an oocyte donor, and of freezing one's eggs are necessarily encountered as everyday life, immersed in the particularity and irreducibility of the present, while also pointing toward the already lived and yet to be lived life.

In seeking to assay this qualitative texture, I draw on another term of Raymond Williams's—"structures of feeling"—which beautifully modulates the loose relationships between formally articulated worldviews, historical dynamics, and "meanings and values as they are actively lived and felt" (1977, 132). Williams writes,

> It is not only that we must go beyond formally held and systematic beliefs, though of course we have always to include them. It is that we are concerned with meanings and values as they are actively lived and felt, and the relations between these and formal or systematic beliefs are in practice variable. . . . An alternative definition would be structures of *experience*: in one sense the better and wider word, but with the difficulty that one of its senses has that past tense which is the most important obstacle to recognition of the area of social experience which is being defined. We are talking about characteristic elements of impulse, restraint, and tone; specifically affective elements of consciousness and relationships: not feeling against thought, but thought as felt and feeling as thought: practical consciousness of a present kind, in a living and interrelating continuity. We are then defining these elements as a "structure": as a set, with specific, internal relations, at once interlocking and in tension. (1977, 132)

"Structures of feeling" suggests useful ways to consider, for example, the anxiety or grief evident in many of the interviews for this study, ways to trace these intense feelings back into public understandings of genetics and historical norms around family formation and the ordering of motherhood, without reducing their particularity and personal force for the woman interviewed. Rather, it provides a way to investigate how the institutions and formal practices of biomedicine and family formation are effective as "lived, actively, in real relationships" and through "a kind of feeling and thinking which is indeed social and material . . . [yet] before it can become [a] fully articulate and defined exchange" (Williams 1977, 130–131). Structures of feeling distill broad social formations in the detail of everyday life, not as derivative phenomena, or "secondary evidence," but as a condensate in an irreducible, yet social, particularity. So while few of the interviewees explicitly articulated their grief, hope, anxieties, and misgivings in terms of genetic research, kinship, gender, or the political economy of household formation, their personal accounts speak directly to these analytic systems and inform our understandings of them in enriching ways.

The lived and felt values around oocytes that emerge from the material are often expressed in terms of fertile *time*: time lost and regretted, time wasted in failed conception attempts, time gained through egg freezing, and the ways in which the experience of fertility recursively redeems or condemns life already lived and life to come. The present management of oocytes through IVF, egg donation, or egg freezing are all ways to order the everyday present into a much desired future, when the woman's biological relations with partner and children would be secured. This temporal inflection of feeling is not arbitrary. Rather it responds to the material capacities and constraints of oocyte biology, their continuity of the germ line, and their time-critical fragility. Women's biological schedules are recalcitrant, and their generative capacities elusive, so that they press on other dynamics in women's lives (education, work, household establishment, partner selection) and make their negotiation more time acute.

In chapters 4, 6, and 7, I explore how this sense of generational integrity and continuity is disrupted by the practices of oocyte donation, in which the donor's genetic lineage substitutes for the recipient's. The sense of indebtedness, obligation, fractured maternity, and anxiety expressed by the women I interviewed toward their anonymous donors constitutes another key element of the structure of feeling generated around the oocyte economy. Oocytes can constitute intercorporeal relationships between women because they can be transferred from one to another, and the quality of these relationships, their meaningful and affective dimensions, is highly informative of the historical dynamics at play in the increasingly global relations of reproduction.

Organization of the Book

The chapters proceed in a loose chronological order, although each chapter also takes a particular thematic focus. Chapters 1 and 2 are the most explicitly historical. In chapter 1, "Temporal Oocytes: Fertility and Deep Time," I consider the evolutionary history of human oocytes, and how their particular material qualities as mammalian gametes shape the ways in which they can be experienced. I foreground three biological characteristics: One is the deep generational continuity inherent in the gametes, their ability to memorialize the evolutionary history of speciation and family ancestry and propel it into the future through reproduction. The second is anisogamy, the sorting of mammalian gametes into tiny, copious, motile ex vivo sperm and large, rare, nonmotile in vivo eggs. Much ART treatment is designed to make eggs more like sperm, ex vivo, numerous and mobile, and hence manipulable in the laboratory and clinic. The third quality is totipotency, the capacity of the oocyte not only to continue the germ line, as do sperm, but also to incite and unfold the embryo and establish the gestational conditions for pregnancy. The demand for donated oocytes is largely driven by this totipotency. For women seeking a reproductive donor, the provided oocytes can establish the elusive pregnancy, while for stem cell scientists, totipotent oocytes can unleash the ontogenic processes that establish a patient-specific embryonic stem cell line. Totipotency then confers immense value on oocytes. Of all the cell lineages, only they can act to establish new lifetimes. For women they can readily become the aspect of embodiment most committed to what I term in chapter 1 "generational time," the succession of lifetimes and the possible ways in which generations are created and coexist.

Chapter 2—"Twentieth-Century Oocytes: Experiment and Experience"— draws on the historical overlap between these two terms to account for the emergence of human fertility medicine from the experimental ethos of twentieth-century reproductive biology. The IVF techniques that would eventually be deployed to treat women with fertility problems were pioneered and refined in laboratories concerned with pure research into mammalian embryology and endocrinology, as well as applied research in livestock husbandry. In both cases the experimental methods involved controlled interventions into the processes of conception and ontogenesis, pragmatic technical tinkering designed to perturb normal developmental sequences and render at least some elements external to the mammalian body so that they could be resequenced and recombined in useful ways. I argue that this more strictly scientific sense of experiment is rendered as a form of self-experimental experience for those women who participate in the drawn-out attempts to apply animal reproductive techniques to human beings. This willingness to be "test-tube women" during the 1960s and 1970s was driven largely by the early successes of the women's movement in improving reproductive conditions, through the advent of the Pill and the rescinding of punitive legislation around the legitimacy of children born out of wedlock. The sudden reduction in adoptable children propelled many women to seek a clinical solution to their fertility problems, so that the inability to have children became a medical rather than a social issue. They, and the clinicians who struggled to adapt techniques developed in livestock to human physiology, discovered that the most obdurate, intractable point in the process involved the production and harvesting of oocytes. At this point, oocytes became objects of direct, discreet experience and desire.

Chapter 3, "Precious Oocytes: IVF and the Deficit Spiral," explores this intractability at length through interviews with women who have gone through IVF, either for their own fertility treatment or as an altruistic donor to another woman. I argue that while IVF and its ancillary techniques are designed to create oocyte surpluses, in practice they create deficits. In vitro fertilization has a repertoire of treatments and techniques addressed to the production and harvesting of numerous ex vivo oocytes. Women who go through such treatments, however, frequently, indeed usually, discover that these techniques cannot compensate for the scarcity and incalculable potency of their oocytes, qualities inherent in the materiality of oocytes that no current techniques can redress. Through a detailed account of the interviewees' experiences, I consider the ways in which the incalculable qualities of oocytes, their resistance to ranking and testing, in concert with their capacity to transmit generational time and to establish gestation, help to constitute their nonfungible value for women in fertility treatment. They are precious, without substitute, and the most fragile point in the quest for a child.

In chapter 4, "Global Oocytes: Medical Tourism and the Transaction of Fertility," I consider the development of a global market for "other women's oocytes," when the bid for a child with one's own does not succeed. Unlike one's own oocytes, with their irreducible qualities of genetic selfhood, kinship, and ancestry, third-party oocytes are ordered on (usually) regional markets and transacted between women with similar appearance and quite different economic positions; that is, older, wealthier women purchase oocytes from younger, poorer women with whom they share a physical resemblance and an ethnic phenotype. These transactions may take place within a single jurisdiction, but the regulatory discrepancies between states has also produced a global market. Women who live in more conservative jurisdictions, like Australia or France, where transaction is criminalized, will travel to more permissive locations to purchase oocytes as part of fertility treatment. In this chapter I examine the experience of nine women based in Australia and the UK who have traveled overseas in their bid for a child. Their experience tells us a great deal about the structure of feeling ordered through the oocyte economy. The decision to travel overseas is generally taken after extended, onerous engagement with fertility treatment, and an intensified desire for fertile oocytes as the means to a child. Though all but one of the women I interviewed did give birth to children, most were haunted by the figure of the oocyte provider, in the sense that they lacked a secure sense of their claim to motherhood proper. They felt, to varying extents, that the provider was the "proper" mother, that the child did not sufficiently resemble them, and that the child might resent them in the future because they were maternal imposters. I discuss what this sense of insecurity says about the public understandings of genetics and about the contemporary constitution of motherhood. I also consider a compelling exception to these accounts, a women of European descent who intentionally sought out a nonidentical "Asian" provider, a strategy associated with "rainbow" adoption and queer family formation among the cosmopolitan denizens of liberal cities like Sydney (Murphy 2013).

Chapter 5, "Cold-Chain Oocytes: Vitrification and the Formation of Corporate Egg Banks," examines the transition from the transaction of fresh oocytes to that of frozen ones. The global market I describe in chapter 4 has developed as a form of medical tourism because all parties to the transaction—provider, clinic, and recipient—have to be in the same place at the same time, for rapid transfer of the fresh matériel. Over the last ten years or so, however, vitrification protocols have been developed to flash freeze oocytes. This technique opens out an entirely new suite of logistical and scalar possibilities for the oocyte economy. In this chapter, based on interviews with clinical and business staff at four egg banks in London, California, and Arizona, I explore how these new logistics reorder both pragmatic and affective relations between oocyte provider and recipient. The intense sense of displacement described by some of the women in chapter 4, the lack of maternal entitlement and deference to the imagined claims of the egg provider, derive, in part, from the one-to-one, batch-by-batch form of the transaction. Each woman has her menstrual cycle synchronized with and receives a complete set of superovulated oocytes from a single provider, and both women have to be present in the clinic on the same day, even if they do not meet. In this sense, the women share different aspects of a single reproductive process, coordinated by the clinic, and this configuration shapes some of the structure of feeling I describe in chapter 4. Oocyte vitrification opens up more modular possibilities, so that transfer is less constrained. Oocytes can be procured without the need for a synchronized recipient. They can be frozen after provision, with batches subdivided into smaller units. They can be shipped through space and kept in time. All these capacities detract from the intense one-to-one nature of fresh transfer. I argue that, just as the subjective experience of blood transfusion changed when blood was fractioned rather than given whole (Waldby et al. 2004; Waldby and Mitchell 2006), so too do oocytes lose some of the personified aura. Rather the role of the provider becomes more professionalized, a development also evident in research donation. I take up this point further in chapter 7.

In chapter 6, "Private Oocytes: Personal Egg Banking and Generational Time," I consider another dimension of vitrification: the development of personal egg banking for women who wish to preserve their own fertility in time. The ethics of private oocyte banking, or "social egg freezing" as it popularly termed, are now much debated, particularly as high-profile companies like Google now offer egg-freezing fees as part of a salary package for young female employees.[9] I want to set this approach aside, however, and consider instead what the desire to freeze one's oocytes says about fertile temporality. The women I interviewed wished to use egg freezing as a way to reconcile otherwise incommensurable time scales, those of credentialing, career, partnering, and household formation on the one hand, and those of generational time on the other. I use the idea of generational time to account for the way that the fertility of oocytes transmits generational continuity, locating the woman in her parental and ancestral lineage and projecting her into the future of children and descent. This capacity is time critical and must be deployed in the first half of a woman's life, a constraint that often conflicts with the demands of professional life and the vagaries of thirty-something couple formation in the metropolitan centers that form the focus of this book. So, private egg banking has gained commercial traction and a clientele because it offers a way to synchronize these different time scales, at least in theory, and tamp down the urgency to conceive.

Chapter 7, "Innovation Oocytes: Therapeutic Cloning and Mitochondrial Donation," moves away from personal experience and considers two of the most salient research programs associated with oocytes: their use to create patient-specific stem cell lines, sometimes termed "therapeutic cloning," and their very new application in clinical treatments to prevent the transmission of mitochondrial conditions from mother to child. While these applications are at one remove from questions of personal fertility, they nevertheless require women to act as oocyte providers, as each program depends on the biological action specific to human eggs. These two domains are highly specialized, and only a handful of laboratories are actively pursuing such research. I examine some of the specific procurement dynamics used in each domain, and analyze what this tells us about how the oocyte provider is figured. In the case of SCNT and therapeutic cloning, the history of procurement is highly politicized, and very few laboratories have succeeded in establishing a sustainable form of provision. I examine two such programs in the United States, which have successfully created highly professionalized provider panels. In the case of mitochondrial donation, only one UK clinic has approval to recruit egg donors, and at present their approach is modeled on that of reproductive donation and appeals to community. Mitochondrial donation returns us to the question of structure of feeling, however, because its regulatory framing separates "proper" genetic motherhood from donor contribution and tries to secure a clear hierarchy between different maternal claims in the creation of the healthy child.

In the concluding chapter, I try to consider what the structure of feeling played out in these pages might tell us about the ethics of oocyte *regulation*, how legal systems might better reflect the new relations of kinship, maternity, and family formation described by the oocyte economy.

One. Temporal Oocytes

....

Fertility and Deep Time

In popular culture, oocytes are biological clocks. Women in the postindustrial democracies are confronted again and again with the irreversible ticking away of their fertility, instructed in the women's health and lifestyle media to seize the day and conceive before the ticking falls silent. This finite clock time is the salient *temporal* experience of fertile time for women. The clock motif recurs again and again in the interviews conducted for this study, as an explanation for the various strategies these women used to manage the conundrum of their fertility. The biological clock expresses an important aspect of fertile time—its finite horizon, its movement toward a vanishing point midway through the lifetime of women in the global north. It conveys only a thin sense, however, of the dense temporal capacities invested in oocyte biology. It foregrounds the most familiar, everyday sense of time, linear, consecutive, regular, a predictable mechanism that moves forward, each discreet point in time superseding the last. The ubiquity of clock time in everyday life means that this sense of time is ready to hand. The ticking clock expresses a certain experience of time as constantly lost, wasted, dissipated, not to be re-gained. In this context, *biological* clock time implies a regular dissipation over the biological life course, a calculable diminution that extends to the time of the calendar, as each successive birthday subtracts another year of possible fertile time. Yet this quite particular organization of everyday time—into minute, regular, passing increments—is rarely adequate to the experience of the life course, with its dolors, renewals, endurable and unendurable stretches, unpredictable intensities, and abrupt reversals. Nor can it encompass the nature of biological time. As Adrian Mackenzie observes in his work on synthetic biology, clock time does not adequately describe the multiple stochastic temporalities of living process. Rather the aim of much contemporary biotechnology is to find ways to articulate the clock time of industrial infrastructures with the qualitative complexity and nonlinearity of cellular and genetic rates: "Growth, reactions, metabolism, signaling, cycles, mutation, catalysis, transcription, translation, recombination, folding, degradation and synthesis are just some of the rates that biology grapples with. Establishing mathematical and experimental control over rates lies at the heart of the engineering of biology" (Mackenzie 2013, 8).

The biological clock time attributed to oocytes is not a straightforward measure of their inherent temporal qualities but rather the outcome of various testing regimes used in fertility medicine to provide clients with a pragmatic indicator of their likely success rates if they undergo various procedures. So rather than treat biological clock time as descriptive, in what follows I want to unpack some of the complex temporal investments and capacities of the oocyte and begin to think about how these capacities shape women's experience of their location in fertile time. While the biological clock idiom has an expressive appeal for many of the women interviewed, it by no means exhausts their sense of the significance of their oocytes, or the ways in which they reach into the past and future. To better account for this significance, we need an understanding of the *thick* time (Neimanis 2014) invested in oocyte biology, a sense of time that includes and accounts for the deep past and indicates the deep future. The term "thick time" evokes the sense in which the entire genealogy of the species and ancestry is played out in the real time of lived life. The present always brings the past with it, so each living being summarizes its own inheritance. Astrida Neimanis writes that "thick time . . . gathers all of the pasts and possible futures within itself. In terms of corporeal generosity, it retains a material memory of the bodies that world its matter in the present. . . . Time is not a path, stretching behind and beyond us. It is not something we are simply 'in,' or which we progress 'through.' We (in the most expansive sense possible) are space-times gathering our pasts and making multivalent futures possible" (Neimanis 2014, 118).

From this point of view, our bodies are archives that memorialize and accumulate their own histories. They prolong the past of the organism in the present and propel the present into the future. This sense of time is quite other to clock time, in that it is explicitly continuous and ramified, rather than successive and discrete. Temporal qualities coexist with one another; they are not jettisoned into the past. The oocyte creates thick time both in its profound conservation of the germ line and mitochondrial DNA, and in its totipotent generation of new organisms, new lifetimes. Since the birth of Dolly the sheep in 1996, biologists can point toward an even more startling temporal capacity of the oocyte, its ability to reverse gene expression and take the genome of a somatic cell back to totipotency. When deployed in laboratory conditions, it can reanimate the embryonic potentials of differentiated, dedicated adult cells. These qualities and temporal possibilities coexist indivisibly within the vitality of oocytes, linking ancient microbial life to the white heat of contemporary biotechnology.

Oocytes and the germ line are only one among many other cell lineages that coincide temporarily in individual human bodies, concatenating and disassembling in gestation, birth, growth, and death. Each cell lineage leads in turn back into evolutionary time. They remind us that the life of subjective experience, of our sense of ourselves as singular, coherent, sensate, and conscious organisms, is built on a whole other substrate of inhuman and prehuman life—cellular, bacterial, ribonucleic, cytoplasmic— that is in a sense outside our experience, *or at least the usual scale of what counts as experience.* In this book I want to address how women experience their oocytes, how they live with them as elements of the self and make sense of them in a quotidian way. Yet I also want to explore the hinterland of biological, material life and deep time that constitute oocytes and consider how this impinges on what they can mean and how they can be lived with. This necessarily involves a consideration of evolutionary biology, and how living matter memorializes its own past and invents its own future through the conservation and elaboration of evolutionary experiments. As beings that necessarily live the scale of their lifetime as embodied time, we partake of the ways our biology *continues us in time* in singular, qualitatively irreducible ways.

While this temporal scale seems elusive, too inhuman and extensive to accommodate the time of lived life, I consider throughout the book how the women who participated in this study evoke what I term "generational time." This is a pivotal term that can account for how experienced time intersects with deep time. This term encompasses the succession of lifetimes and the possible ways in which generations are created and coexist. The women interviewed for this study often expressed a strong sense of indebtedness to the family that precedes them and to the family that they hope to create, to both past and future generations. While this sense is circumscribed by the immediate generations, the parents and grandparents at most, it was expressed often as the only possibility of both a happy proximate future, in the creation of a child, and of an extended legacy, a line of descent. The oocytes were considered essential elements in the ways the women could position themselves in the time of successive lifetimes.

Generational time also suggests the more intensive sense of *generative* time, the time of fertility, sexuality, conception, gestation, birth, of the biological relations of reproduction. As I explore in the following section, oocytes continue the germ line, the cell lineage with the most direct form of continuity through biological time, lived through the reproduction of each new generation. Notably, Henri Bergson, the great philosopher of time, singles out the germ line for its qualities of continuity, its particular memorization of the life of previous and future generations in its conserving and ontogenic capacities:

> This current of life, traversing the bodies it has organized one after another, passing from generation to generation, has become divided amongst species and distributed amongst individuals without losing anything of its force, rather intensifying in proportion to its advance. It is well known that, on the theory of the "continuity of the germ-plasm," maintained by Weismann, the sexual elements of the generating organism pass on their properties directly to the sexual elements of the organism engendered. . . . *Life is like a current passing from germ to germ through the medium of a developed organism.* It is as if the organism itself were only an excrescence, a bud caused to sprout by the former germ endeavouring to continue itself in a new germ.

The essential thing is the *continuous progress* indefinitely pursued, an invisible progress, on which each visible organism rides during the short interval of time given it to live (Bergson and Mitchell 1911, 27; emphasis in the original).

In relation to human reproduction, men and women "ride" their fertile capacities in markedly different ways. For men, the life of their gametes tracks their life course more extensively, but for women in the developed world, their capacity to create a new generation is confined to the first half of life. When combined with the social asymmetries of mothering responsibility, this necessarily affects the way women experience their inclusion and agency in generational time, rendering it more acute as it accelerates toward its vanishing point. This constraint is more urgently felt because of the difficulty of reconciling it with the liberal sense of time as "the passage towards complete actualization" (Colebrook 2009, 11; Neimanis 2014), as an instrumental medium at the disposal of the entrepreneurial subject who maximizes the accumulation of human capital (Becker 1993). This is the time of career, with its (hopefully) upward ascent and aggrandizement. As Claire Colebrook suggests, this instrumental time is one of *self-generation* and liberal individualism, a time which is both implicitly masculine and unable to acknowledge the indebted, imbricated, and relational time involved in the reproductive transition from one generation to the next. She writes, "Man is that animal who has no nature, essence or being other than the form that he gives to himself, and history and generations are merely the matter through which man creates himself" (Colebrook 2009, 11). This irreconcilable quality, banalized as work-life balance, propels women into an expanding field of reproductive consumer services—contraception and ovulation management, egg and embryo freezing, sperm purchase, in vitro fertilization (IVF) and the various techniques of ART—to manage the intersection of multiple temporalities in our bodies.

Mammalian Sex

The gametes—oocytes and sperm—are essential elements in the biological architecture of mammalian sexual reproduction. In the history of biology, human gametes have been persistently attributed with qualities derived from the social organization of gender—active sperm, passive egg, and so on—a practice that has been ably critiqued by feminists (e.g., Martin 1991; Keller 2000). The point of this critique is to demonstrate the teleological reasoning in biology that works backward from existing gender arrangements to their functional analog in living processes. In what follows, I do not want to further develop this kind of critique per se, but rather consider how we can understand the human gametes, and particularly the oocyte, as a cell lineage that materializes the deep time of microbial life and its innumerable contingencies.

That is, I want to first think about the temporality of the oocyte as a *cellular* temporality, with dynamics and qualities specific to this level of scale. Drawing primarily on the account of cytobiology developed by Lyn Margulis and Dorian Sagan, I want to consider to what extent the powers and constraints of oocyte biology are shaped by deep time. Gamete life and organism life coincide imperfectly, and gamete life is driven by constraints and possibilities often more proper to microbial life in general than to the interests of human life specifically. As Margulis and Sagan put it, "The private activities of early cells are involved even today in the courtship of human beings. The intimate behaviour of single cells has simply been elaborated to include animals and their behaviours and societies. Mammalian sex is a late and special variation on a far more general theme. . . . Human sex is almost identical to that of some of the protistan microbes" (Margulis and Sagan 1986, 2).

Gametes are first of all cells. Cells are the minimum unit of life in Margulis and Sagan's terms, because all are autopoietic (they metabolize their environment) and all reproduce, in the sense that they *replicate* themselves. Nucleated cells (e.g., somatic cells in animals) are diploid, with two sets of chromosomes that reproduce themselves by splitting and doubling, or mitosis. The history of life on earth has been primarily one of mitotic self-replication, where reproduction involves an increase in the number of individual entities, without mixing the genetic contribution of two or more parents. Mitotic division is the form of reproduction characteristic of bacterial and amoebic life, in which very rapid increases in number (in for example the plasmodium microbe that causes malaria) can be generated from a single parent cell through replication of its DNA and division of nuclei and cytoplasm. Mitosis is also how multicellular organisms grow and develop into entities with differentiated types of tissues (e.g., contractile cardiomyocytes in the heart, hepatocytes in the liver), as cellular material replenishes itself through division. Mitosis is the mechanism of organism growth and development.

The gametes, however, involve a process that Margulis and Sagan term "meiotic sexuality," which implicates at least two parental entities. The gametes are haploid cells, with a single copy of chromosomes; they create the conditions for the process of meiosis, which involves fertilization, the recombination of chromosomes from each parent to reconstitute a complete, yet unique, genome for the resultant zygote. This process is a familiar account of how mammalian and human conception takes place, but Margulis and Sagan defamiliarize it by locating the processes in the dynamics and constraints of the earliest microbial life, demonstrating the ways in which fertilization and embryogenesis, in humans as in other multicellular species, is a response to the microbial ecologies that make up cellular life. Or to put it another way, "In some organisms [including humans] . . . a certain kind of two-parent sex became intimately connected to reproduction because of events occurring in the ancestral phyla" (Margulis and Sagan 1986, 15).

In their account, meiosis was an innovation in the early history of microbial life (700 million years ago) that dramatically increased the rates and kinds of differentiation available to organisms, and hence their adaptability to changing environmental pressures. In its earliest form, it involved the differentiation of single-cell organisms which reproduce through mitosis (the prokaryotes) into two-cell organisms (the eukaryotes). In the two-cell eukaryotes, the ancestors of all multicellular life, one cell retains mitotic capacity and the second cell can only reproduce meiotically. This combination gives the various kinds of genetic material in the cell (mitochondria, chromosomes) far more scope to express as organism variation, and to transmit and conserve developments. It also solves the problem of species reproduction combined with differentiation and specialization of tissues, because the gametes retain a transmittable copy of the intact heterologous genome, whereas the nucleus in the somatic cells can modify or lose organelles in the process of differentiation. All contemporary animals retain this mutually exclusive organization of cells, so that unlike all other tissues in the body, the gametes cannot reproduce mitotically but must proceed through fertilization.

In most animals and plants, the necessity of routing reproduction through the process of meiosis and fertilization means that "the sexual cycle . . . returns each generation to a single cell: a zygote with organelles such as mitochondria and plastids derived from the female parent" (Margulis and Sagan 1986, 173). This is the pivotal moment in larger biological regulatory processes to ensure the reproduction of species populations and the retention of what Margulis and Sagan term "the master set of genomes" for a species, the germ line, the set of cells that become the gametes. "The fundamental constraint of development . . . is the obligatory nature of the retention throughout development of the entire set of genetic possibilities in at least one cell lineage in good working order and capable of continued growth and cell reproduction. . . . All eukaryotic individuals must reserve, in a form capable of continued reproduction, their genetic components, the remnant bacteria in the combined form of the nucleocytoplasmic, mitochondrial, plastid and undulipodial genomes" (Margulis and Sagan 1986, 175–176).

The gametes, then, are not simply the cells that create the conditions for ontogenesis, the beginning of each individual life, they are also the cells that link past generational time with future generational time. They route the life of each generation back through its initial conditions as microbial, single-cell life, so that each zygote is both the terminus and the beginning of a cycle of generational time. At the same time, the path from meiosis in ancient phyla to mammalian and human sex is not a teleological ascent to higher and higher degrees of functionality but rather a contingent, blind probe process in which innumerable accidental experiments are conserved in the cell lineages. In the gametes, mitochondrial DNA, transmitted only by the maternal germ line through the oocyte, is postulated to descend from oxygen-metabolizing microbes that became symbiotic in the eukaryotic cell (Margulis and Sagan 1986, 69). The tail of sperm, which gives them their characteristic motility, might have developed in symbiosis with spirochete bacteria, and all sperm have tails with a similar structure, from those of water ferns to those of men (Margulis and Sagan 1997). Nevertheless, while the process is an accumulation of contingencies and constraints, meiotic sexuality is, in effect, the engine of complex life, the force that acts through time to proliferate species. As Elizabeth Grosz puts it, in her reading of Darwin and evolutionary time,

Sexual difference is the very machinery, the engine, of living difference, the mechanism of variation, the generator of the new. Sexual difference ensures that each individual is unique, irreplaceable, new, historically specific, different from all others, and able to be marked in relation to all others. Without sexual difference there may be life, life of the bacterial kind, life that reproduces itself as the same except for contingency or random accident, except for transcription errors at the genetic level, but there can be no newness, no inherent direction to the future and the unknown. (Grosz 2011, 101)

The gametes roll up in themselves the deep history, or memory, of sexual reproduction as continuous experimentation and proliferation, its debt to and perpetuation of inhuman life. They organize the continuity of generations, the movement from parents to offspring, as well as the generation of difference between parents and offspring, the production of a perpetual instability and open-endedness to the reproduction of the future.

Anisogamy and the Ovarian Reserve

So we can see that oocytes, as the gametes particular to women, bring with them particular capacities, constraints, and qualities that link women's bodies to an evolutionary history of meiotic sexuality, and more proximately to the reproductive biology of other mammals. In women's encounters with fertility medicine, one particular set of constraints is salient: anisogamy, the difference between small, motile ex vivo (after ejaculation) sperm, and large, nonmotile, in vivo eggs, and its corollary, the parsimony that reproductive endocrinologists term the "fixed account," or ovarian reserve.[1] Anisogamy is a quality of almost all contemporary multicellular creatures. As Paul Cox (2011) notes in his introduction to a collection of papers on anisogamy, there is no clear advantage over isogamous (similar size) gametes, and the explanations for gamete dimorphism are various and contested. As a quality that has evolved innumerable times in various lineages it represents a "robust evolutionary solution" (Cox 2011, 4), yet the set of contingencies or constraints that continually produce dimorphism are not clear. Cox suggests that anisogamy is no more functional than isogamous gametes, but rather that each assortment establishes certain kinds of environmental stability with particular sets of evolutionary advantages and disadvantages. Margulis and Sagan propose dimorphism as a form of cell specialization, which reflects the difficulty of combining the qualities of motility, necessary for the gametes from different parents to find their way to each other, with the necessity to provision the zygote, so that it has a sufficiently nutritious environment in which to grow. Tiny sperm, all nucleus and little cytoplasm, can become motile because they jettison mass, while large ova can accumulate mass because they are stationary: "As long as the equality of the parental nuclear contributions is maintained, division of labor leads to efficiency: one parent cell stores food and stays put and the other loses all its excess baggage and moves around" (Margulis and Sagan 1986, 195). The oocyte provides not only the nuclear components from the maternal parent but also the mitochondria and other organelles shed by the sperm in the process of spermatogenesis and the acquisition of motility. The oocyte also provides cytoplasm, considered as simply passive nutrition for the zygote in much of the twentieth-century history of biology, but now recognized as a crucial element in the dynamic of gene interaction and expression that guides embryogenesis (Keller 2000). These elements make the oocyte such a large cell, among the largest in the mammalian body.

A further constraint pertains to the degree of expenditure involved for the organism in the production of gametes. Cox (2011) argues that biomass is axiomatic: "Each reproductive individual has only a fixed biomass available for gamete production, and so the greater number of gametes produced, the smaller those gametes must be" (Cox 2011, 12). This constraint is particularly suggestive when trying to think about the specificity of mammalian and human oocytes. In the biology of mammalian gametogenesis, not only the size but also the process of production is asymmetrical. Spermatogenesis in humans initiates at puberty and continues until death, although the viability of sperm themselves decreases with age. In men with normal levels of fertility, sperm are produced in a continuous process at a rate of 1,500 per second, and healthy ejaculate contains at least 39 million sperm (Cooper et al. 2010). As only one sperm is required for fertilization, we can see that spermatogenesis involves a high degree of redundancy. The process of oogenesis in mammals is also proliferative, but at a much earlier point in the process. The stem cells that produce primordial oogonia in the female fetus are extinct in most mammals by the time birth takes place. The numbers of primordial follicles, the structures that generate mature oocytes after puberty, are set in a fixed account, or reserve, of 10^6. This reserve is subject to various forms of attrition and selection so that the development of mature oocytes, the form of cell necessary for meiosis, is decidedly parsimonious. While follicles are recruited in their hundreds during any given menstrual cycle, only one will mature for ovulation while the rest succumb to atresia. "In a typical woman, who cycles 13 times per annum between the ages of 13 and 50, less than 0.1% of her follicles will have shed oocytes by the time of menopause" (Faddy and Godsen 2003, 44).

The Biological Clock

This oogenic parsimony shapes the way fertility is available to women as a capacity of their bodies. The attrition of primordial follicles begins before birth in girls, and by puberty, with the onset of ovulation, most follicles have already been lost. The rate of loss accelerates with age, and below a certain threshold of primary follicles, ovulation ceases with menopause. Hence human oocytes are biological rarities, and the body's capacity to produce them dissipates across the first half of the life course. This dissipation was expressed by many of the women interviewed for this study as "lost time," an expenditure of fertility that could not be regained or reversed. This metrical understanding of oocytes is not entirely artifactual, as suggested, I think, by menstrual (in the sense of monthly) logics, the way in which women's ovulatory systems count out the phases of the moon and the cycle of the year. Yet this intuition is sharpened by fertility research (like that cited above) devoted to precise calculation of dissipation rates over the life course of populations, and by various testing regimes that calculate the levels of the ovarian reserve in individual women. (I discuss this relationship in detail in chapter 6.) In each of these forms of calculation, we can discern an attempt to link the biological time of oogenesis and ovulation with the predictability of clock and calendric time. This linkage is pragmatic for fertility medicine, as clinicians and bench scientists seek methods to estimate a woman's chances of pregnancy through IVF or other forms of assisted reproduction.

For many of the women who turn to fertility treatment, these techniques offer a solution to the problem of coordination they face when trying to reconcile the desire for children with the demands of working life. They experience the ticking of the biological clock because it occupies the same temporal terrain as their career and credentialing process—the time of industry, production, the working day—the time that never seems sufficiently extensive to include reproductive time. The biological clock is an idiom that enables calculation in the same currency as forms of professional time. It also involves a certain kind of gestalt, in which the ticking clock of fertility partakes of the ticking clock of mortality, the time of life as unceasing, irreversible, metrical dissipation. In this scenario, fertile oocytes seem to have miraculous powers to redeem time, to put a new lifetime in train, which will revalue all the time that precedes it. They have the powers of ontogenesis, the creation of a new individual from the immortal substance of the germ line. With the advent of mammalian cloning, they also have the powers to reverse the developmental pathways of the organism, taking differentiated cells back to their embryonic totipotency. In this sense, fertile oocytes could be described as the antithesis of clock time, working backward against the irreversibility of time's arrow, to undo the biological aging process, to dedifferentiate the adult somatic cell and the adult organism and return it to its moment of zygotic potential. To these timescales, I now turn.

Totipotent Time

"It is the egg, rather than the sperm, which holds the key to [life's] transmission between the generations" (Short 2003, 9). This claim, made by an obstetric clinician, reflects recent reevaluations of the asymmetrical powers of the gametes in the biology of embryological development. These reevaluations have been driven by the resurgence of cell biology, the expanded practices of reproductive medicine, and the success of mammalian cell nuclear replacement, or cloning, in the late twentieth and early twenty-first centuries. Each of these fields has contributed to an appreciation of the complexity of oocyte biology, and particularly its capacity to unfold the process of ontogenesis, the creation of entire new organisms.

In this they depart from the mainstream of twentieth-century biology, the "century of the gene," as Evelyn Fox Keller describes it (Keller 2000), dominated by molecular biology and a commitment to nuclear DNA as the causal agent in biological organization. This approach treats gene action as the key to the process of fertilization, cell differentiation, and embryological development, which as Keller, Susan Oyama, and others note (Kay 2000; Keller 2000; Oyama 2000), privileged the sperm's nuclear contribution over that of the cytoplasmic oocyte. In their respective accounts, the bioinformatic nature of much genetic practice has shored up a reductive analogy between the gene and the computer program, where the gene acts as the master program, delivering instructions to the cytoplasm. The basis for this code-centric formulation was posed by Francis Crick in his now notorious central dogma paper, "The Biological Replication of Macromolecules" (1957), in which he states that the flow of information in genetics is always unidirectional, from gene to protein. Genes, he asserts, are the origins of form, the repositories of instructions for morphogenesis, and are unaffected by their environment. "Once information has passed into protein it cannot get out again," he states (Crick, cited in Kay 2000, 174).

In formulating gene action in this way, Crick and the majority of classical molecular geneticists reinscribed an ancient form/matter distinction, datable at least to Aristotelian biology, in which form is the principle of masculine activity impressing itself on passive, feminized matter in the process of reproduction (Oyama 2000). Here, the feminist argument runs, the central dogma of classical genetics denies the possibility of complex, multilateral exchanges between genes, cytoplasm, organism, and environment, and privileges the tiny sperm, all nucleus, over the large oocyte, with its many organelles and large complement of cytoplasm. James Bonner's work on the genetic program (Bonner 1965), for example, proceeds on the unspoken assumption that the cytoplasm of the egg in conception plays no role in the transmission or regulation of inheritance. Hence the nucleus *must* be the locus of biological activity, the site of the genetic program for development, and sperm cells are composed almost entirely of nucleus. Keller comments, "The conviction that the cytoplasm could neither carry nor transmit effective traces of intergenerational memory had been a mainstay of genetics for so long that it had become part of the 'memory' of that discipline, working silently but effectively to shape the very logic of inference" (Keller 2000, 85).

This gene centrism has more recently given way to more epigenetic accounts of embryogenesis that foreground cellular dynamics and demote the gene to but "one of several protein events, that can be reversed, mimicked and reengineered," as Sarah Franklin puts it (2007, 34). Such accounts are far more attentive to the oocyte's contribution and to the role of complex feedback mechanisms and emergent dynamics between maternal and embryonic cells. In Margulis and Sagan's account, for example, the large cytoplasmic oocyte is the locus for symbiotic cooperation between organelles (nuclei, plastids, mitochondria) and dispersed kinds of gene products, as well as its quantum of DNA, and it is the cell that ensures the transmission of these various forms of biological information to the offspring. The interactions between these various communities, plus the nuclear contribution of the sperm in the process of cell fertilization, regulate the development of the resulting zygote (Margulis and Sagan 1986).

In more mainstream developmental biology, the fertilized oocyte is now widely acknowledged to direct the early stages of embryogenesis, while also exercising more long-term effects on the offspring (Tadros and Lipshitz 2009). The mechanisms within the oocyte accomplish what is termed the "maternal-to-embryonic transition" (MET), the period of zygotic and embryonic development prior to the implantation of the embryo in the endometrium. During this period, the developmental trajectory of the embryo is governed by maternal genetic information found in the proteins and RNA in oocyte cytoplasm. The embryo gradually recruits this information to its own genome.

To briefly describe this transition: At the point of fertilization, both the sperm and oocyte genomes are inactive, and for the embryo to develop, they must be activated and remodeled by proteins in the oocyte cytoplasm (Latham 1999). The oocyte integrates the maternal and paternal haploid genomes into the unique diploid genome of the new organism and sets the processes of embryogenesis and gestation in motion. According to a recent textbook account of oocyte biology:

> The first developmental function of an oocyte is to transform both paternal and maternal genomes into a single totipotent functional genome. Although the genetic information is brought by both gametic genomes at fertilisation, it is now clear that epigenetic modifications that take place during the first cleavages [mitotic divisions of the cells] affect both early and late developmental events. All the changes in nuclear envelopes and chromatin proteins necessary to the formation of the embryonic genome are performed by maternal factors present as proteins or mRNA in the oocyte cytoplasm. This cytoplasm also ensures the time-regulated activation of the embryonic genome . . . neither too early, because it would result in the random expression of genes . . . nor too late, because zygotic transcripts have to take over the maternal transcripts and proteins (Duranthon and Renard 2003, 100)

In other words, the oocyte not only synthesizes the embryo's unique genome, it also modulates the sequence of gene interactions so that they proceed in an orderly way. The early embryo's capacity to transcribe (that is, express) its own genetic material emerges incrementally from maternal transcription, and at any point during the MET, maternal and embryonic versions of the same transcript can coexist (Tadros and Lipshitz 2009). Gradually maternal genetic information is inherited by the early embryo, and the steady reduction in maternal mRNA (i.e., messenger RNA, which mediates between DNA and protein production) is thought to act as a "maternal clock," influencing the mitotic cell division cycle of the early embryo (Tadros and Lipshitz 2009). Cytoplasm inherited from the oocyte continues to modify gene expression, not only during early embryonic development but also in fully differentiated, mammalian adult tissues. Moreover, recent experiments with nuclear replacement in mice suggest that alterations in gene expression can be inherited through the germ line (Roemer et al. 1997), so that "maternal factors have long term and even trans-generational effects" (Duranthon and Renard 2003, 101).

During the period of maternal-to-embryo transmission, then, the cells of the zygote and blastomere (four-cell division embryo) are an indivisible complex of maternal and embryonic material. This is the period of "totipotency," when each cell has the capacity not only to differentiate into the various tissues in the organism, but also to establish the organism as a whole, and to create the uterine conditions for its existence. These cells set out the initial division into an inner cell mass, which becomes the body plan of the organism, and the outer cell layers, which establish the trophectoderm, the placental membrane which creates the conditions for gestation (Mitalipov and Wolf 2009). Totipotent cells, as the term implies, are attributed with the highest possible degree of biological potential, in the sense that they can give rise to the highest degree of complexity and to the *organization* of both the organism and its conditions of development. Degrees of potential are understood to be surrendered as each stem cell travels along a path of further differentiation in the developing organism; from totipotency, to the pluripotency of embryonic cells, able to generate almost all the individual tissue types in the adult body, although not the organism itself; to multipotency, able to produce particular cell lineages (so hematopoietic cells give rise to the various blood cell types, but not to cardiac cell types); to unipotency, where stem cells only differentiate into one type of tissue (for example, epithelial skin cells). All these classifications of potential retain the self-renewing capacity specific to *stem* cells, but in this system, potential and potency is lost as each cell lineage travels along a path of greater differentiation and dedication to particular cell types (Melton 2014).

Until fairly recently, this linear path toward dedication was understood to be nonreversible, in part because of an overestimation of the role of genes in the fate of the somatic cell. The process of differentiation into specialized cell types was understood to be the result of nonreversible gene expression. Once cells were programmed to produce a particular kind of cell, they lost their ability to produce different kinds of cells (Keller 2000). As Franklin puts it, "Differentiated cells were defined on a scale of irreversible temporality; they could not . . . revert to a pre-specialised state in which their fate was open-ended" (Franklin 2007, 41).

This view of gene action and cell temporality was upended by the birth of Dolly the sheep (Gottweis, Salter, and Waldby 2009). In 1997, Ian Wilmut and other scientists from the Roslin Institute in Scotland announced the first successful birth of a mammal, Dolly, conceived not through the process of fertilization, but rather through a technique known as somatic cell nuclear transfer (SCNT). Popularly described as cloning, SCNT is a technique of particular interest to this study, because it is organized around the epigenetic capacities of the oocyte and demonstrates its biological and ontological flexibility.[2] It involves the creating of an embryo through the in vitro insertion of the nucleus of a somatic cell from a donor into an unfertilized egg. The oocyte has in turn been enucleated, that is, had its own nucleus removed to make way for the introduced nucleus. The oocyte is then able to reactivate the totipotency of the donated material, effectively returning it to its zygotic status and rerunning its developmental trajectory.

Scientists at Roslin had successfully created SCNT sheep prior to Dolly, using embryonic cells to provide donor nuclei. Dolly's birth, however, generated far more attention from life scientists (and the world's media) because the donor cell was taken from the cryopreserved mammary tissue of a six-year-old Finn Dorset ewe (Franklin 2007). That is, the donor cell was a fully adult, fully differentiated form of tissue. Drawing on a decade of experience with reproductive cell cycle research, Wilmut and his team introduced the adult nucleus into eggs taken from Scottish blackface sheep. The oocytes took the nuclear material back to its totipotent state, effectively returning the adult cellular material to its earliest moment of existence and greatest potency. The resulting embryo was introduced into the uterus of a surrogate mother, who carried it to term, producing Dolly, a genetic copy of the by-then-long-dead Finn Dorset ewe. In the notice announcing her birth, Wilmut and colleagues dryly summarized the significance of their innovation:

> The lamb born after nuclear transfer from a mammary gland cell is, to our knowledge, the first mammal to develop from a cell derived from an adult tissue. . . . Birth of the lamb shows that during the development of that mammary cell there was no irreversible modification of genetic information required for development to term. This is consistent with the generally accepted view that mammalian differentiation is almost all achieved by systematic, sequential changes in gene expression brought about by interactions between the nucleus and the changing cytoplasmic environment. (Wilmut et al. 1997, 813)

The birth of Dolly provoked extensive reevaluation of received wisdom about gene action; tissue differentiation; the idea of linear, clocklike biological development; and most important for this study, the significance and capacities of the oocyte. The technique of scnt demonstrates the extent to which oocytes are the master (or perhaps mistress?) cells that preside over the process of ontogenesis, able not only to unfurl the life of the zygote and direct it toward its multicellular adult future, but also to take adult, multicellular organisms back to their initial conditions.

Fertile Temporalities

We can see from my brief treatment that oocytes contain the most complex possibilities of any form of cellular action. They orchestrate multiple kinds of temporality in their ability to unfurl new living beings and to reverse the aging process of cellular life, resetting its totipotent possibilities. These rich temporal and generative capacities give oocytes a pivotal position in the assisted reproductive process and lend them much clinical and scientific significance. Women who wish for children, and who seek reproductive medical assistance, may also have to come to terms with the refractive, elusive, and often incalculable generative capacities of their oocytes as their means toward the child.

In the next chapters of this book, I examine the ways in which women experience and value their oocytes, and the kinds of temporal and social relations oocytes enable and constrain. These include the creation of children, but they also extend to many other forms of relationships and senses of continuity or discontinuity, as well as different senses of value. For stem cell researchers, the possibility of creating patient-specific stem cell lines through a form of human SCNT is the highest aspiration of regenerative medicine. Regenerative medicine is a new medical discipline that aims to reverse the aging process and other forms of senescence and degenerative pathology through the regeneration of tissues—for example, neurological tissue lost in Alzheimer disease, or cardiac tissue lost through infarction—rather than through organ transplant. While some forms of regenerative method depend on stimulating the patient's own tissues (autologous tissue), others involve transplanted stem cell tissue from a donor (allogeneic tissue), using the renewing capacities of pluripotent and multipotent stem cells (Mason and Dunnill 2008). As I have argued in several papers, the regenerative medicine method seeks to redistribute the cellular potency of the maternal-embryonic relation from generative to regenerative ends, revivifying the health of aging populations through transplantation of stem cells derived largely from women's reproductive tissues (embryos, cord blood, fetal cells, menstrual blood; Waldby and Cooper 2008, 2010; Cooper and Waldby 2014). Here we can see systematic attempts to leverage the singular temporal capacities of women's reproductive biology to renew life, diverting it to clinical applications that seek to remedy the aging process. This capacity too has become an element in the experience of fertile duration, as women negotiate the obligations and demands placed on their biology by the clinical possibilities of regenerative medicine.

Two. Twentieth-Century Oocytes

....

Experiment and Experience

Oocytes have a capacity to orchestrate complex, nonlinear biological temporalities in the longue durée of mammalian history. In this chapter, I locate oocytes in a more proximate history, one that describes the ways in which oocytes have become objects of explicit experience. As an element of most women's reproductive biology, they necessarily form part of their general experience of fertility, part of the gestalt of womanly embodiment as the life of the gametes assert themselves in the more general life of the body. This assertion is lived as distinctive moments in the feminine life course—menarche at adolescence, the lunar cycle of menstruation, the moments of conception, the longueurs of pregnancy and parturition, and the disconcertions of menopause in middle age. The material qualities and particular capacities of oocytes play out in these moments, and as we are all immersed in the duration of our biological life, we cannot *but* experience these qualities as the givens of existence.

Nevertheless, I would argue that there is a more specific history in which oocytes become *discrete objects of desire and experience*. Over the course of the twentieth century, as the biological sciences extended their knowledge of cellular and molecular life and became more tightly tied to national medical and industrial priorities, oocytes were gradually objectified as cell lineages with particular capacities and potential applications. Prior to this historical moment, their capacities could not be separated out from an integrated experience of reproductive physiology as an everyday bodily gestalt, in which tissues and organs cooperated in the "coordinated ensemble . . . [that] comprise[s] the total organism" (Canguilhem 2008, 17). While their *cooperation* produced fertility (or its absence) as particular kinds of thematizable experience, marked and organized in virtually all cultures, these elements themselves were not ready to hand as experienced, remaining in their opaque, in vivo milieu as a tacit texture.

Nor could we refer to an oocyte *economy* under these conditions. Like other tissue economies (Waldby and Mitchell 2006), the idea of an oocyte economy is that they have a specific therapeutic or industrial productivity that can be ordered in different ways. While they remain in the web of hormonal and physiological interactions in their given biological milieu, they support the life of the organism. Tissues can be ordered into hierarchies of value only once they can be isolated in some way—through interventions that single out and modify their operation in vivo, or through their removal and circulation beyond the organism. Ex vivo tissues can be donated, to sustain the life and health of recipients (for example, blood and organ donation), they may be banked for future use (for example, cord blood), or they may become elements in laboratory research (for example, embryonic stem cell lines). In each case, tissues are procured, managed, banked, and circulated in a system designed to maximize their latent productivity. Tissue economies are not simply technical matters, because the ways in which human tissues are procured and distributed involve fundamental social questions about power relations (who donates to whom, under what circumstances, with what regulatory protections?) and social values (what do particular tissues mean and how do they count to donors, recipients, research facilities, commercial biomedicine?).

In what follows, I explore the historical conditions through which oocytes became objects of both experience and economy. Throughout the course of the twentieth century, oocytes became *experimental* objects, as the reproductive sciences tinkered with their functions, capacities, and potentials. This experimentation was driven to a considerable extent by public investment in *reproductivity as a form of industrial production*, as a capacity underpinning food security, population health, national defense, and postwar prosperity. While experimentation was initially focused on livestock gametes as leverage points in the agricultural sector of national economies, the ethos and knowledge were incrementally transferred to human gametes as the century progressed. Meanwhile, over the course of the twentieth century, but particularly after the 1960s, women adopted an experimental approach to their own bodies, to the constitution of their fertility, and to the limits of femininity through the optic of feminism (Murphy 2012). When these two domains of experimentation intersected, oocytes gradually emerged both as discrete objects of desire and as objects with *scarcity* value, amenable to ordering, hierarchy, and transactions of various kinds.

In making this claim, I am working from George Canguilhem's proposals regarding the circular relations between experience and experiment in the life sciences, how one translates into the other (Canguilhem 2008). His account of these relations elaborates on the historical etymology developed by Williams (1983), which I describe in chapter 1, where the term "experience" conveys a sense of both subjective empirical knowledge and scientific inquiry, a relationship more evident in French, in which the word *expérience* may be translated as variously to encounter, to experience, to discover, and to test.

Canguilhem works from this double significance to argue that knowledge of organs and tissues cannot be established outside experimental methods. The life sciences tinker with the constitution of an organism's internal milieu, interventions that modify vital norms, rather than study them passively. At the same time, the experimental life sciences are systematic forms of the experiential knowledge that is necessarily generated by all living beings. He writes, "For us, there exists a basic kinship between the notion of experiment [*experience*] and [biological] function. We learn our functions over the course of experiences and our functions then become formalized experiences. And experience is first and foremost the general function of every living being, that is, its debate with its milieu. Man first experiences and experiments with biological activity in his relations of technical adaptation to the milieu" (Canguilhem 2008, 9). In this kind of approach, the reproductive sciences and developmental biology, with their interest in the generation of new organisms and the processes of inheritance and generational transmission, share common ground with feminism and women's interests in modifying and expanding the scope of their embodiment. Both share a focus on addressing and changing certain kinds of reproductive limits and identifying new kinds of reproductive potentials, even as the knowledge generated in the reproductive sciences could be (and was) deployed in ways that women found oppressive. In this shared experimental space, oocytes crystallize as experiential objects, as women in the 1970s and 1980s are prepared to risk new, untried assisted fertility techniques in their capacity as moral pioneers, forging new approaches to the negotiation of ethical issues and risk assessment (Rapp 1987).

In Vivo Oocytes and the Problem of Mammalian Reproductive Biology

The gametes, eggs, and sperm became objects of twentieth-century biology as leverage points in a broader project to gain technical traction on the processes of reproduction. Each had a long history within the biological sciences as objects of inquiry and philosophical speculation. Early Enlightenment science, with its interest in the physiology of generation and the identification of fundamental life processes, produced systematic studies of reproduction: William Harvey's *De Generatione Animalum* (1651), Reiner de Graaf's comparative studies of the ovaries in the 1670s, Anthony van Leeuwenhoek's descriptions of sperm enabled by the newly invented microscope (1677), and Karl Ernst von Baer's illustrations of the mammalian egg in *De Ovi Mammalium* (1827).

These anatomical studies became more dynamic in the late nineteenth century, as the field of embryology emerged from the broader evolutionary reconfiguration of biology. The developmental processes of embryos, and their comparative study across various species, were compelling fields for biologists interested in testing and refining the grand insights of evolutionary theory. The ways in which embryos acquire tissue specialization, morphology, and species-specific features were regarded as keys to the understanding of human and animal origins (Hopwood 2000; Morgan 2009). The idea of development itself, of the progressive unfolding of form, guided the nineteenth-century embryologists' interest in demonstrating biological life as a sequence of steps through which the organism moves (Hopwood 2000; Oyama 2000). In the process of identifying developmental trajectories through systematic collection of embryos, turn-of-the-century embryologists also adopted a more interventionist attitude to reproductive biology, the kind of systematic modifications to living process that Canguilhem argues is the modern biological method (Canguilhem 2008). If embryology described a developmental sequence with identifiable steps, then each step offered a potential insertion point for techniques designed to delay, accelerate, divert, or resequence living processes. In Franklin's history of IVF, she notes that fin de siècle embryology treated the embryo, and the process of conception, as mechanisms, and hence open to other, experimental, mechanisms:

> Much of the experimental work in experimental embryology was . . . philosophically motivated, while at the same time becoming more boldly instrumental in disrupting natural trajectories and inventing, or forcing, new recombinant ones. New microsurgical tools and techniques were developed as part of an expanding culture of . . . experimentalism based on the transfer of substances between whole organisms in order to study the parts of organisms, or to create new mosaic organisms that were deliberately designed to be different from what would emerge normally. This newly interventionist embryology enabled mechanical parts of embryos to become tools of investigation to understand, or probe, the causal dynamics of morphogenesis, reproduction, regeneration, development, and heredity. . . . Naturally existing forms and substances were increasingly viewed as biological mechanisms that could be imitated, inverted, reassembled, reverse engineered, or otherwise manipulated. (Franklin 2013, 115)

While the embryological work of Wilhelm His, Ernst Haeckel, and Walter Heape was primarily directed to settling debates in evolutionary theory, their experimental techniques lent themselves to more pragmatic interests. As Franklin (2013) notes, Heape's development of the basic model of embryo transfer, in 1890, set the parameters for all subsequent studies of mammalian reproductive biology, because it set out a method for experimentation with in vivo reproduction. Embryology in the late nineteenth century, and indeed in the twentieth century, had focused on amphibians and marine animals because their habits of ex vivo fertilization made them easier to study (Bavister 2002). Heape conducted an experiment that diverted the process of mammalian fertilization out of one body and into another. He recovered two fertilized ova from an Angora rabbit and transferred them directly to the fallopian tube of a hare that had been fertilized by another hare three hours beforehand. The hare eventually gave birth to four hares and two Angora rabbits (Biggers 1991).

For Heape, this experiment was designed to demonstrate the sovereignty of the gametes in the transmission of traits, and the lack of hereditary contribution from gestation. In the process, however, he had invented a method through which mammalian reproductive biology could be both studied and modified as a living system, and it was to be adapted to multiple ends. Embryo transfer, and the protracted quest to fertilize mammalian oocytes ex vivo, were two techniques that underpinned the pragmatic twentieth-century desire to *industrialize* the germ line. Here I am following the work of Adele Clarke (Clarke 1998, 2007), who demonstrates how principles of scientific management, Taylorism, and industrial production became the mission of the reproductive sciences. This industrial vision developed incrementally from the experimental ethos of nineteenth-century embryology, in that it depends on regarding reproductive biology as a sequence of step-like processes that can be disassembled and reassembled, as well as engineered in different ways. Such an engineering approach can readily communicate with business models of industrial scale and capitalist efficiency (Cooper and Waldby 2014).

In the field of agriculture and livestock husbandry, biological life was framed through this mission as a latent force of production, a source of economic and social potentials that should be reordered and placed at the service of national priorities and commercial interests. The reproductive sciences sought to make the processes of animal conception, ovulation, spermatogenesis, embryogenesis, gestation, and lactation more closely resemble those of twentieth-century mass manufacture, with more predictable input and output measures, standardized components, and clocklike rates. If biology could be managed more efficiently, it would be possible to introduce economies of scale into agricultural production, producing greater yields and fewer losses, and make reproductive processes more predictable and open to further technical configuration (Clarke 2007, 330). Jean-Paul Gaudillière comments that these new techniques form part of "a more general search for bio-productivity" in the mid-twentieth century, "which equated the management of both human and animal with industrial husbandry. The culture of standards and homogeneity inherited from the factory model of scientific management and rationalization was in this perspective as, if not more, important than the technical capacity to increase yields, that is, to deliver more numerous, less fragile and more rapidly growing newborns" (Gaudillière 2007, 525).

The field of reproductive science was composed of a heterogeneous set of players and disciplines, particularly in British and Australian embryology, U.S. endocrinology, and various porous mixtures of medicine, biology, and agricultural and veterinary sciences. While progressive farmers in Australia, the United States, and the UK had developed techniques during the nineteenth century for selective breeding as a method of livestock improvement, generating greater milk yields, wool production, and so forth (Franklin 2007), the reproductive sciences sought ways to directly manipulate the cellular and endocrinal processes of conception and gestation, to eliminate the vagaries of opaque in vivo reproduction and replace it with the efficiencies of the laboratory and the factory.

These efforts had their initial successes under the auspices of artificial insemination (AI). Techniques for preserving and transporting bovine semen were worked out during the 1930s, to inseminate large numbers of cows dispersed across different small herds and thereby improve herd exposure to high-yielding bulls. Gaudillière (2007) notes that in Britain, AI was treated as a public service, organized through a network of publicly funded centers where veterinary scientists could select the best bulls and exercise centralized control of the insemination of herds, treated effectively as one national herd. The technique was designed to as a way to improve genetic stock qualities and synchronize aspects of milk production, aims that became more urgent under conditions of war mobilization in the 1940s. It delivered veterinary scientists, farmers, and the British state far more detailed control over herd reproduction because it changed both spatial relations and biological ratios. It permitted insemination without direct physical contact and scaled up both the number of inseminations from each unit and the distribution of units across geographical space. While under natural conditions a bull could fertilize thirty to forty cows per year, by 1947, using AI, one bull could fertilize five hundred to one thousand cows a year (Clarke 1998).

Oocytes too were reorganized in the twentieth century along industrial lines, although they proved less tractable than semen, and their management involved much more protracted experimentation. Mammalian eggs were only slowly adapted to experimental methods, as they were difficult to maintain in vitro. Oocyte research was focused on in vitro fertilization, as a method to both study the basic science of mammalian development and gain traction over the most potent point in the reproductive cycle, the point where each generation of animals is rerouted through its single-cell origins. It was also focused on the *temporality* of the egg; the material obstacles to both animal and human IVF revolved around the difficulty of reconciling the highly species-variable, yet exquisitely specific, cellular schedules of oocyte maturation and fertilization with the clock time of laboratory and hospital schedules.

Warren Lewis and Paul Gregory's remarkable cinematic approach to the developing egg was a signal moment in the history of this research. In 1929, Lewis and Gregory, of the Carnegie Institution, Washington, DC, the leading U.S. center for embryology research, obtained newly fertilized eggs from three rabbits and filmed their division, from the initial cleavage stages to the eight-cell blastocyst stage. Using microphotography and stop-frame exposures twice per minute, they documented the process of early mammalian development in a form that could be animated, that is, sped up, so that the emergence of embryonic form can be presented to the viewer in a time scale more suitable for general appreciation than the actual duration over several days. Stop-frame exposure also enables the viewer to slow down, reverse, and replay particular sequences, inspecting moments one by one. Lewis and Gregory used this novel control over the time of embryogenesis to publish a detailed account of early embryological development (Lewis and Gregory 1929), and their method became popular among embryologists. Indeed, a later work of embryological cinema, Alan Beaty's *Inovulation*, was to inspire the young Robert Edwards and set him on the path to mouse embryology and eventually to human IVF (Edwards and Steptoe 1980). My broader point, however, is that Lewis and Gregory's film was a major innovation in the project to represent the process of fertilization and blastocystic development as a linear sequence with a specific temporal order, which could potentially be reordered and rerun differently. In this sense they realized the bid of reproductive biology to treat embryological development as a *bestand*, a standing reserve of potentials and utilities (Heidegger 1977), and a sequence that could be reconciled with the regularity of clock time (Waldby 2000).

While Heape had established the model system for mammalian embryo transfer in the 1890s, IVF could not be reliably performed in mammals until the mid-1950s, despite many prior attempts and indeed claims of success, most notably those described in Gregory Pincus's study *The Eggs of Mammals* (1936). Biologists were focused on IVF as a way to make mammalian embryology as transparent and readily studied and manipulated as that of species with ex vivo eggs. As Barry Bavister puts it in his history of early IVF,

> The progress of research was hindered by the internal site of mammalian fertilization, which means that events involved in fertilization of mammalian eggs and early embryonic development cannot be investigated readily in their natural environment. Therefore, information concerning the relationship between the egg or the developing embryo and the immediate maternal environment is difficult to obtain. . . . Information can be derived much more readily from the study of eggs that are fertilized and then develop in vitro. Not only can the process of fertilization be closely observed, but also factors contributing to normal and abnormal fertilization and development can be examined. The progress of fertilization or embryogenesis can be frequently, if not continuously, observed and the conditions of culture can be varied to examine their effects on development. Thus, a wealth of information is available from studies in vitro, given the technical ability to accomplish them. (Bavister 2002, 182)

The discovery of sperm capacitation by Min Chang and Colin Austin in 1951 was a pivotal point in the establishment of repeatable IVF procedures; that is, the discovery that sperm required a set amount of time in the female reproductive tract before they were capable of fertilization (Bavister 2002). By 1954, this discovery enabled in vitro fertilization of rabbit eggs, but the complete, verifiable demonstration of mammalian IVF did not take place until the late 1950s. Min Chang, at the Worcester Foundation, Boston, successfully fertilized rabbit eggs in vitro, cultured them to cleavage point, transferred them to gestational mothers, and demonstrated that they developed normally into live young with the characteristics of their genetic parents (Chang 1959).

Bavister argues that this demonstration, the many subsequent repetitions and adaptations of Chang's procedures to other mammals (mice, rats, sheep, dogs), and the birth of healthy young over a period of fifteen years opened the way for embryologists and clinicians to consider the application of IVF techniques to human reproduction. Nonetheless, the development of human IVF, and the elaboration of an oocyte economy, were not simply technical dynamics in a progressive trajectory from rabbit to human reproduction. Rather, the long experimental path leading to routinized human IVF gathered up in itself several social tributaries. These include the twentieth-century change in the status of the child, the deregulation of the Fordist family, the resurgence of feminism in the late 1960s and 1970s, and the elaboration of an experimental approach to reproduction and to the capacities of the feminine body, particularly around the reversal of shame.

These social dynamics propelled women into often heroic participation in experimental IVF during the 1970s. Hence, practitioners in the two leading clinics, in Melbourne, Australia, and Oldham, UK, could refine and tinker with human fertilization until its opacities and synchronies could be rendered into predictable steps, ratios, and procedures. In particular, they had to identify the specific time signatures that characterize human oocytes, their rates of maturation, and the precise stages in the unfolding of fertilization, the zygote, and the blastocyst to move toward live birth. This research demanded a generous supply of ex vivo oocytes. Later, clinical experimentation to produce actual pregnancies also depended on the procurement of ex vivo oocytes, a hazardous enterprise for fertility patients, and a laborious and fraught task for clinicians. The first generation of IVF births in the late 1970s and early 1980s were only possible because women were prepared to treat their own bodies as components of experimental in vitro systems, and to enter actively into the process of tinkering, trial and error, repeated failure, partial success, and incremental adjustment that this involved. They were truly, to use the language of the time, test tube women. In what follows, I consider the social relations of reproduction that propelled the experimental phase of IVF and the emergence of an oocyte economy.

The Desire for Children and the Medicalization of Infertility

The attempts during the late 1960s and 1970s to adapt animal IVF to humans were to some extent driven by scientific ambition, particularly the desire to be the first team to produce a health IVF baby. They were also a clinical response to shifting social dynamics around the organization of the family, the value placed on children, and women's changing civil status. During the late nineteenth and early twentieth centuries, older, communal approaches to infant care, particularly baby farming and wet nursing, and the pursuit of large families as a source of household labor and income, were displaced by social arrangements that favored women having fewer, more precious children. With the abolition of child labor and the newly universal obligation to educate children, family size reduced. Many of the substantive arguments for women's suffrage revolved around the need for better maternal care of children, as an effect of improved civil status and women's education (Waldby 1983). One of the goals of early twentieth-century child welfare organizations was to strengthen and sentimentalize the mother-child bond, to enshrine it as a private and singular relation, and to sacralize children as emotionally priceless, rather than as sources of additional labor for the family economy (Zelizer 1994). As Viviana Zelizer notes, this process of cultural valuation meant that childless women were somewhat stigmatized, and in the United States and elsewhere, commercialized forms of adoption sprang up to capitalize on new, sentimentalized demand for desirable types of children—healthy, beautiful infants. Infertility hence emerged as a personal problem under these conditions, but solutions were sought through the brokerage of orphaned or surrendered children, rather than through medicalization.

By the 1960s, however, these social methods began to fragment, as both feminism and civil liberties movements improved women's civil status, and unmarried women in particular gained greater social recognition and control over sexual relations. In Australia, the supply of adoptable children contracted as single motherhood shed some of its social stigma with the passage of the Births and Deaths Registration Act (1960), which legitimated children born outside wedlock and allowed single women to keep their babies. The advent of the Pill, in 1961, and the decriminalization of abortion in various states in the late 1960s and early 1970s, meant that women had far more control over their fertility, and the number of extramarital births dropped precipitously between 1970 and 1976 (Carmichael 1996).[1] In the United States, the same dynamics reduced the number of white babies available for adoption throughout the 1970s (Zamostny et al. 2003). In the UK, from 1970, single women were far more prepared to undertake single motherhood than had been the case in the early twentieth century (Kiernan, Land, and Lewis 1998).[2]

Hence, the favored types of adoptable children, the healthy beautiful infants that feature in Zelizer's analysis, became scarce, replaced by fewer children forcibly removed from situations of neglect and abuse. Adoption became onerous and less and less likely to result in a child free from class disadvantage, so women with sufficient means increasingly consulted gynecologists in the hope that some medical procedure might restore their fertility. This willingness to turn to medicine also partook of the broader transformation of human reproduction precipitated by the advances in hormonal pharmacology and culture techniques already described, the propagation of population-control strategies by the World Bank and family planning organizations, and feminist advocacy and self-help. As Michelle Murphy puts it, in the second half of the twentieth century, sex and reproduction became more technically and socially malleable, and more politically contested than in earlier eras:

> With the aid of synthetic hormones, immortal tissue cultures, and delicate pipettes the very biological processes of human fertility, and even the sexual form of the body as male and female, became profoundly manipulable. . . . Large scale national and transnational schemes encouraged the technological limitation of births, distributing birth control pills, IUDs, and surgical sterilization to millions, helping to alter the fertility of entire populations for the sake of a greater economic good. . . . This rapidly emerging technical ability to alter human and non-human reproduction, stretching from molecular to transnational economic scales, was accompanied by new promises for the politicization of life—not just should, but *how* could reproduction be transformed? (Murphy 2012, 1)

Murphy uses this general historical transformation to investigate a specific response to the new malleability of reproduction: the feminist self-help movement, which encouraged women to investigate and understand their sexual health and reproductive possibilities through the formation of self-help groups, women's health centers, and the publication of manuals like *Our Bodies, Ourselves* (Boston Women's Health Book Collective 1973). While the explicit politics of feminist self-help is somewhat at odds with the preparedness of infertile women to volunteer for experimental gynecological procedures, I would nevertheless argue that both practices worked to bring women's reproductive biology into thematizable experience through experimentation. In each case, women were prepared to confront existing systems of moralization that worked to exclude the biology of femininity from awareness and to shame it. The difference between the two fields was that feminist self-help was a strategy to render in vivo experience thematizable through analytic and critical discussion

(Lemke 2011), particularly a critique of medical hierarchy itself, while women's participation in IVF research was more individualized and more beholden to the authority of the clinician. Moreover, feminist self-help was primarily concerned with limiting fertility, with *contra*ception, while IVF was explicitly and directly concerned with *con*ception. At the same time, their involvement partook of the larger question at stake: How could reproduction be transformed? Could the reproductive capacities of their bodies be reordered through laboratory systems to create healthy children? They were to discover that the answer to that question largely depended on the development of clinical ability to manipulate their eggs.

Experimental IVF and the Lineages of the Oocyte Economy

As more and more women presented themselves to gynecology practices for fertility treatment during the late 1960s and 1970s, the problem of infertility acquired more prestige within the profession, and clinicians were interested to identify promising lines of research that might point toward new treatments (Leeton and Riley 2013). The research field in the late 1960s and early 1970s was largely confined to animal work, so the beginnings of human IVF involved collaborations between embryologists experienced in mammalian IVF and gynecologists with surgical skill and large numbers of infertile patients prepared to lend their bodies to experimental biology. Two sets of collaboration led experimental IVF: that among embryologist Robert Edwards, gynecologist Patrick Steptoe, and nurse Jean Purdy, based at Cambridge and Oldham District General Hospital in the UK, and among embryologist Alan Trounson and obstetricians Carl Wood and John Leeton at the Royal Women's Hospital and the Queen Victoria Hospital in Melbourne, Australia.

Both Edwards and Trounson brought extensive experience with mammalian oocyte harvest and IVF to bear on the difficulties of human IVF. In Edwards's case, his research was initially carried out in mouse reproduction during the 1950s at Waddington's Institute of Animal Genetics in Edinburgh. His dissertation concerned the effects of modifying chromosomes on embryonic development, using AI techniques. His initial foray into oocyte work was motivated by the unsociable hours dictated by murine estrus cycles. After months of working at night to synchronize AI with ovulation, he collaborated with his fiancé and fellow student Ruth Fowler and U.S. colleague Alan Gates to treat mice with gonadotrophins to stimulate ovulation "during office hours" (Edwards and Steptoe 1980). Their success with timed ovulation and successful gestation was initially met with skepticism. The understanding at the time was that only immature ovaries could be stimulated with gonadotrophins, and that mature ovaries were unresponsive. Edwards was quick to appreciate the multiple potential applications of this technique for agricultural animals and human infertility. He and Steptoe note the "perfect synchrony" of the eggs as they responded to stimulation, "like setting accurate alarm clocks" (Edwards and Steptoe 1980, 33). Examining the ova under a microscope, they see the precise choreography of the maturing oocyte, the rearrangement of the chromosomes, and the formation of the first polar body. Edwards writes, "Because of the regularity of these events, we could predict all the ripening stages of the mature egg: where the [chromosomal] manoeuvres would be at a particular time, when the eggs were ready for ovulation and fertilisation. Would the timing be the same in farm animals and in human eggs? I wondered, once more thinking of the practical applications of such knowledge" (Edwards and Steptoe 1980, 33). Edwards embarked on a research program to characterize the synchronic possibilities of human oocytes: Would they mature in culture? At what rates and under what hormonal circumstances? To move into human research, however, required a steady supply of research eggs and involved the complications of working not with a ready supply of sacrificable mice under laboratory conditions but with human patients under hospital conditions. He carried out this characterization work on abandoned ovarian tissue, excised during surgery for polycystic ovarian disease and ectopic pregnancy, first at Edgware General Hospital in London and later at Johns Hopkins Medical School.[3] After several years of research, Edwards was able to produce a timetable for human oocyte maturation, cross-tabulating the age and medical condition of the donor with the precise time intervals taken for each oocyte to move through its developmental program: "After the release of the human oocyte from its graafian follicle, meiosis is resumed in vitro and is completed to the stage found at ovulation in vivo, i.e., metaphase II and first polar body. The oocytes mature synchronously even though taken from ovaries in widely different endocrinological states, so that the stage of development after a particular duration of culture can be predicted with accuracy" (Edwards

1965, 929). He concluded that this predictable developmental sequence, which moves forward in vitro as well as in vivo, meant that human in vitro fertilization had to be possible, in the same way it had been possible with other mammals. Moreover, the administration of hormones to the woman could increase the rates of oocyte production and hence chances for IVF pregnancy (Edwards 1965). For Edwards, the stage was now set to move the research to human experimental participation; that is, to identify a hospital population prepared to go through experimental procedures so that the techniques of human IVF could be worked out.

While Edwards was focused on moving his research into the clinic in the UK, Alan Trounson was beginning his research on oocyte physiology as a master's degree student in the Department of Pastoral and Wool Sciences at the University of New South Wales, Sydney. His aim was to identify factors that produced multiple births in sheep, a topic with considerable economic significance in Australia, where the wool industry was the mainstay of the national economy. His work involved developing techniques for embryo transfer and bench research on ova physiology. In the early 1970s he began to work with Neil Moore, head of the Department of Animal Husbandry at Sydney University who had a research program focused on IVF in ewes, based at the McCaughey Memorial Institute in Jerilderie, western New South Wales (NSW). Like Edwards, Moore and Trounson produce precise time tables of in vitro development, cross-tabulating types of culture medium and hormone administration, with hours elapsed for each stage, and with live births of lambs, as well as experiments to divide ova and culture blastocysts (Moore 1970; Trounson and Moore 1972, 1974; Trounson et al. 1974). Trounson was certain that the key to understanding the processes of in vitro fertilization and embryology in all mammalian species lay with the complexities of the egg, and this formed the main focus of his research. In an interview with Trounson in April 2014, he told me, commenting on this early work in ewes,

> So the focus was, if you like, on the egg. So here I'm asking questions
> about . . . the nature of the egg and the ovary, and I went to do my PhD at
> Sydney University with Neil Moore, who I was doing those experiments
> with, because I found the whole area of embryo transfer fascinating. So
> again, I focus back on the egg because it was . . . to me, driving a lot of
> the components around animal reproduction, so if you were collect-
> ing eggs, you could make embryos and so on. . . . So, the sperm was

coming in, but it was kind of peripheral in my view, as something that was added to, if you like, the mixture, but it was essentially the egg which was really dominant as the life form. It was the one that was progressing through generations. It was the one that had the mitochondria that transferred on. . . . The sperm seemed to be there to mix up the genes a bit and provide for variety in offspring rather than anything else.

Trounson finished his doctoral dissertation "Studies on the Development of Fertilized Sheep Ova" (Trounson 1974), and took up a postdoctoral position at Cambridge, funded by Dalgety Holdings, a pastoral industry company. The Unit of Animal Reproduction and Biochemistry, an Agricultural Research Council Unit at Cambridge University, was at that time one of the most advanced centers for ova research in the world. Trounson focused on comparative embryology and the developmental physiology and endocrinology of ova from various livestock species—cows, horses, sheep—and some rabbit work, developing expertise in cryopreservation and culture media and gaining an appreciation of the specificity of oocyte physiology and early embryological development across different species.

Experiment and Experience
Test Tube Women

The period from the late 1960s until the births of IVF babies Louise Brown, at Oldham hospital in 1978, and Candice Reed, at Melbourne Royal Women's Hospital in 1980, involved intensive work to adapt the procedures of animal IVF to infertile women. In 1968 Edwards teamed with Patrick Steptoe, a gynecologist who had pioneered the use of laparoscopy as a safer, less invasive method of surgery than laparotomy, and with better possibilities for egg retrieval. They also enrolled the expertise of Jean Purdy, a nurse, whose dedication not only to the care and welfare of patients, but also to the orderly operation of laboratory procedure and systematic records proved crucial to their eventual success (Cohen, Alikani, and Franklin 2015).

They set up a research laboratory at Oldham hospital to begin systematic experimental IVF work. Initially their work was conducted using abandoned tissue, as they harvested surgically removed ovarian material and attempted various ways to fertilize the eggs. After repeated failures, they found a successful culture medium, originally developed by Edwards's student Barry Bavister to facilitate IVF in hamsters. They published the results of their study in *Nature*, carefully documenting and timing the fertilization of eighteen oocytes from an initial collection of fifty-six (Edwards, Bavister, and Steptoe 1969).

Despite the extremely dry, technical format of the paper, and its modest claims, they suddenly found themselves the object of intensive, overwrought, and worldwide media coverage that revived Aldous Huxley's account of technological birth in *Brave New World* and focused on the dystopian associations of "test tube babies" (e.g., Shuster 1969). This response was in fact a stock narrative, dating back to the 1920s in media coverage of Gregory Pincus's and J. B. S. Haldane's work, and in the broader public imagination about the reproductive sciences and the utopian and dystopian possibilities of "ectogenesis" (e.g., Laurence 1936).[4] The publication of such a well-verified and potentially repeatable study in *Nature*, the journal of record, ignited an energetic response precisely because it was a well-rehearsed theme.

Among the readership for this article was Carl Wood, foundation chair of obstetrics and gynecology at Monash University, in Melbourne. Wood, like many in his profession, was focused on finding treatments for women's infertility as the number of patients increased, and he teamed with John Leeton, an experienced laparoscopist, to establish an experimental IVF program at Queen Victoria Hospital, which had a "steady supply of infertile patients" (Leeton and Riley 2013, 4). In the same year, 1970, Neil Moore, Alan Trounson's supervisor at Sydney University, contacted Wood to tell him about their ovine IVF program and to encourage a dialogue. They met that year at the Australian Society for Reproductive Biology Conference, and Wood visited the Jerilderie research program to study their laboratory methods and protocols. Wood attempted to recruit Trounson to be his laboratory director, but Trounson declined in order to take up his postdoctoral fellowship at Cambridge (Cohen et al. 2005). Nevertheless, Wood was able to assemble a large clinical and research team focused on the development of human IVF. For the first two years, the research was primarily focused on the collection and characterization of oocytes harvested from surgery, as the laboratory staff gained experience in culturing and handling (Kannegiesser 1988).

The two groups, in Oldham and Melbourne, were now poised to begin clinical treatment, to try to foster in vitro fertilization, not only as an experimental method but as a way to create viable blastocysts and establish viable pregnancies and healthy newborns. The move from human IVF research to human IVF treatment was in effect a move from work on *abandoned* ovarian tissue to work on *identified* ex vivo oocytes. The term "abandoned tissue" has a specific legal and moral significance here, expressive of the *lack of value* that this material was thought to have for the patient who provided it. Historically, hospitals and clinics have treated human tissues excised during surgery as freely available for research, without the need for explicit consent from the donor. The patient was understood to have relinquished it, and to have no intention of reclaiming it (Gottlieb 1998). It was tacitly considered to have no value or significance for them, to be waste tissue belonging to nobody (*res nullius*). Hence, it could be legally claimed for research, which added value to what would have otherwise been waste (Waldby and Mitchell 2006). While both teams developed technical expertise using many hundreds of abandoned oocytes, it is unlikely that the infertility patients who provided the materials were explicitly aware of the fate of their oocytes, and we can gain little insight into what meaning, if any, this process represented for the anonymous donors. The status of identified oocytes in clinical treatment, however, is radically different, for all parties. Here we can see how oocytes acquire intense desirability and scarcity value, both for clinicians and for the women whose hopes ride on successful egg retrieval and fertilization. This hope for a child propels many women into demanding and quite risky experimental participation.

No social scientific research documents the experience of women in the ten years of treatment experimentation—roughly 1970 to 1980—leading up to the birth of the first IVF babies. It is possible, however, to infer some of this experience from the accounts written by the key medical players. More recently, Kay Elder and Martin Johnson have conducted detailed investigations of research notes discovered in Edwards's papers at Bourn Hall Clinic pertaining to this period (Cohen, Alikani, and Franklin 2015; Elder and Johnson 2015a, 2015b), supplemented with one former patient interview and interviews with three members of former staff. I also draw on a small amount of fieldwork conducted in the years immediately after those initial successes.

In the case of the Oldham group, Edwards, Steptoe, and Purdy orchestrated an intermediary stage between the use of anonymized abandoned tissue and clinical treatment. For a period, prior to the establishment of proper sterile surgical conditions, they experimented with laparoscopic egg retrieval, to compare those ripened in vivo with those in vitro.

The laparoscope was a crucial technique for the move into clinical work. While abandoned tissue was excised from the body surgically, and hence was by definition ex vivo, clinical work demanded the retrieval of a *particular patient's* oocytes, and their careful laboratory management in the interests of eventually establishing a pregnancy. Laparoscopy combines visual access to the ovaries using a small camera with precise surgical manipulation of tissues, using instruments introduced into the abdomen through small incisions. It has many applications in gynecology, but in this context, it was used to aspirate mature oocytes from the ovarian follicles, so that they could be transported safely from the woman's reproductive tract into the laboratory.

The Oldham team hence began to approach patients to request their participation in stimulated cycles, to gain control over the timing of ovarian maturation, followed by laparoscopic retrieval and attempted fertilization with the partner's sperm. Edwards writes, "So now we had to involve patients in our work. We had to ask Patrick's infertile patients, those desperate for help and willing to undergo many trials in the hope of one day having their own babies, to cooperate in a project that was still in its stumbling early stages. . . . We both agreed that their hopes must not be raised unjustifiably, and that they fully understood their situation—the opportunities and dangers, and how they would be involved" (Edwards and Steptoe 1980, 88). They found, somewhat to their surprise, some patients at least were keen to volunteer, prepared to undergo repeated laparoscopy if necessary. They established a routine with two to three patients a month and tests with different culture media to try to cultivate five-day blastocysts, the point they thought optimal for introduction into the uterus. The detailed archival investigations by Elder and Johnson evidence Steptoe, Edwards, and Purdy's careful approach regarding the experimental nature of their work at this point and their efforts to be honest and transparent with their volunteers. The first 159 laparoscopic cycles, on ninety-seven patients, did not progress to embryo transfers, as the team focused on refining their technique (Elder and Johnson 2015a). Elder and Johnson identify correspondence and minutes that set out the procedures designed to ensure patients were properly informed, and their interviews with the former patient and staff corroborate the sense that patients were aware that they were experimental subjects rather than clinical patients at this point (Elder and Johnson 2015b).

Nevertheless, after the Oldham team eventually succeeded in creating embryos, they were confronted with their patients' feelings when, in the absence of sterile clinical conditions, the embryos could not be implanted. Steptoe was uneasy but simply informed them that the blastocysts represented another step in progress toward human IVF, and the patients are presumed to have accepted this. Edwards, commenting on the patients' preparedness to undergo such emotionally and physically taxing research, notes, "They were totally aware of the medical situation and of what we were trying to do. Several of them were women doctors, doctors['] wives, or nurses, well able . . . to evaluate our methods" (Edwards and Steptoe 1980, 109). In an account of the patients involved with the Monash IVF attempts, historian of medicine Harry Kannegiesser also notes the preponderance of medical and technical backgrounds (Kannegiesser 1988). This suggests a trust in biomedical progress and a personal investment in the benefits of research among at least some of the patients. In one particularly notable case, a thirty-six-year-old woman presented to the Monash team in 1973 with blockage of the fallopian tubes, requesting that the tubes be surgically repaired. She and her husband were told about the experimental IVF program as an alternative treatment, and they elected to participate, in part because they were familiar with similar techniques used on their dairy farm. Their treatment resulted in a short-lived pregnancy, the first in the program history. While the pregnancy did not succeed, it nevertheless proved that an IVF zygote could implant in the uterus, and the news was duly reported in *Lancet* (De Kretzer et al. 1973).

It seems plausible then to suggest that the willingness of at least some patients to undergo often onerous procedures with little hope of personal result arose from a shared experimental ethos, and a preparedness to directly embody experimentation, to make themselves test tube women. At the same time, Elder and Johnson note, the impression of former Oldham staff interviewed for their study was that even when the experimental nature of the treatment was clearly explained, patients participated because they hoped that eventually they might benefit and have the much desired child. Moreover, as female patients in a northern English town at that time, not all were well educated, and staff sometimes felt doubtful about what some patients understood and to what extent they were motivated by wishful thinking (Elder and Johnson 2015b). As I explore in the next chapter, this ambivalence, between properly informed consent and profound hope, continues to structure patient experience of IVF today.

Between 1972 and 1978, both groups attempted numerous IVF treatment cycles intended to lead to actual conception, rather than as a means of optimizing techniques. In Melbourne thirty to fifty patients each year undertook IVF, not as research subjects but as intending parents: that is, they participated under surgical conditions that would allow any successful conception to progress (Kannegiesser 1988). In Oldham, the notebooks reveal that 282 patients in all underwent 457 cycles; 1,361 eggs were harvested over 338 cycles; 1,237 were inseminated, 220 embryos were created, and 112 transfers performed (Elder and Johnson 2015a). Steptoe's patients were disappointed again and again, as pregnancies failed to establish. Edwards describes this disappointment: "What a long slow haul [the patients] had to endure—the initial wait in hospital, the injection of hormones to stimulate the ripening of their eggs, then the laparoscopy, followed by more and different hormones that would prepare the womb to be receptive. And after all that, and after tests to see if they were pregnant, the going home to a house generally without children's voices in it, going back to where they had set out in hope and returned in disappointment" (Edwards and Steptoe 1980, 133). The Oldham group decided that the stimulated cycles seemed incompatible with the establishment of a pregnancy and attempted IVF using a natural cycle. The viability of this approach depended on Steptoe's capacity to retrieve the single egg matured in the ovary, without the scheduling made possible by the predictability of stimulated cycles. Lesley Brown was the second patient to try this approach, and with the help of a new hormonal test to identify the time of ovulation, and a military level of coordination and synchronization among the theater and laboratory staff, Steptoe managed to aspirate a single egg. It fertilized, the pregnancy took, and in 1978, Louise Brown was born, amid a frenzy of British and international media. A second birth, Alistair MacDonald, followed in 1979.

In Melbourne, the Monash group deduced that the British success was based on a natural cycle, and in 1980, using the same approach, they announced the birth of the world's third IVF baby, Candice Reed, at Melbourne Royal Women's Hospital. Reliance on natural cycles was not a sustainable method of clinical IVF, however, as ovulation time was incompatible with hospital time. The collection process might take place any time during the day or night, so theater and laboratory staff were permanently on call, and surgeries could not be booked ahead of time. IVF remained an unpopular activity among administrators while it made such difficult demands on hospital routines.

At this point Alan Trounson's expertise in the modulation of mammalian cycles became crucial to the establishment of IVF as a viable, repeatable treatment, rather than a singular medical novelty. Appointed as Wood's laboratory director in the late 1970s, he went about adjusting ratios, hormone dosages, timings, and cultures to tip procedures in ways more compatible with human reproductive physiology. In 1981, the Monash University team introduce hormonal stimulation cycles using human pituitary gonadotrophin (HPG) and clomiphene as a way to both increase the number of mature oocytes for harvest and control the timing of ovulation and oocyte collection (Cohen et al. 2005). The production of multiple oocytes facilitated the fertilization of multiple embryos, which could be frozen for later use if the current round of IVF was unsuccessful. The technique benefited women whose infertility was caused by fallopian tube problems but could make little difference to women whose problem stemmed from the oocytes themselves. Once oocytes could be harvested and handled in a laboratory, however, they could also be transferred from one woman to another. In 1983, the Monash group established that a woman with ovarian failure could sustain a pregnancy with an in vitro embryo, created using a donated oocyte (Trounson et al. 1983). Prior to this development, gynecologists had assumed that the age of the uterus was also a factor in the difficulties of late conception and pregnancy, but now the way was open for older women to use IVF, if an oocyte provider could be secured.

Conclusion

With these innovations, the basic procedures that underpin human IVF were in place by the early 1980s. The industrialization of the gametes in the livestock sciences had generated techniques to rationalize and manage human gametes at a clinical level. Oocytes were now entities that could be manipulated ex vivo, produced in multiples, and fertilized under the controlled conditions of the laboratory. Their biological schedules could be synchronized with hospital time tables so that IVF could be rationally administered. The oocytes could be transferred between women. Fertility became a capacity detachable from a particular woman and able to be redistributed, so that it was more symmetrical with the qualities of male gametes. These are the initial conditions for an oocyte economy, a system for desire, valuation, significance, transaction, fungibility, and circulation. In the next chapter I draw directly on the experience of women who have undergone IVF treatment, as either a fertility patient or an oocyte donor, to begin to describe the contours of the contemporary oocyte economy.

Three. Precious Oocytes

....

IVF and the Deficit Spiral

The historical trajectory of oocytes, especially in the last century, led to them becoming discrete biomedical objects, open to various kinds of manipulation and management. In this chapter, I consider their status as experiential and social objects, from the point of view of women undertaking IVF. This status is considered implicitly in the previous chapter, in the sense that I discuss the conditions under which women volunteered as test subjects during the fraught ten years leading up to the first successful IVF births. Much of this test experience was organized around oocyte production and retrieval, as was the experience of the first women to give birth to IVF babies in the late 1970s and early 1980s. In this chapter, however, I want to *foreground* the experiential aspects, and particularly the ways in which women come to *value* their eggs as they gain more direct experience of the IVF process.

This gradual valorization may have precursors in their knowledge about women's fertility more generally, particularly if, as is usually the case, they have come to IVF after a history of failed conception attempts.

They may be aware of the notion of the "fertility cliff," for example, a statistical analysis that demonstrates that the probability of conception falls away sharply after the mid-thirties. It has its origins in mathematical modeling of the rate of loss of ovarian follicles (the biological structures that produce oocytes), which shows accelerated exponential loss after the median age of thirty-seven (Faddy et al. 1992). While familiarity with this analysis was largely restricted to endocrinologists and other fertility specialists over the last twenty years, it has recently been propagated into women's popular media and sex education, in part by the fertility medicine sector (Fidler and Bernstein 1999; NSW Ministry of Health 2013; Public Health Association of Australia 2013).[1] Demographers, women's health professionals, and fertility clinicians have expressed growing concern about women deferring pregnancy as they acquire credentials and professional experience and establish stable households, only to find that they cannot conceive because of the age of their eggs. So, for example, one state-based regulator in Australia, the Victorian Assisted Reproductive Treatment Authority (VARTA), in coalition with women's health organizations, conducted a public education campaign throughout 2014 entitled *Fertility is Ageist*, designed to raise awareness among women of the age-related decline in fertility (Victorian Assisted Reproductive Treatment Authority 2014). It has become something of a topic du jour in the women's print media and the supplements page of the daily press (see, for example, Twenge 2013; Ellen 2014; Healey 2014; Tran 2014), particularly as public fascination with "social" egg freezing has quickened. (I discuss this particular twist to the oocyte economy in chapter 6.)

So women in developed economies at least are more and more likely to be somewhat aware of the peculiar, truncated time line described by their oocytes, "the most rapidly aging cells in the body" (Trounson and Godsen 2003, frontispiece). Nevertheless, demographic forces—extended credentialing, the cost of household establishment, the extension of the life course, and the iterative nature of heterosexual relationships—all push women to later childbearing. They cannot or do not wish to deploy their fertility when it is abundant, because it conflicts with the other demands on their time and labor, irrespective of their knowledge about fertility decline. Hence, many women, needing to establish economic security in high-cost cities like Sydney and London, hope that deferred childbearing will be possible. If they find that their ability to conceive dwindles steadily in their thirties, many will turn to IVF.

In vitro fertilization, in turn, is organized around the procurement of multiple ex vivo oocytes. The chances of successful conception depend heavily on the number and fertility of the oocytes that can be obtained as an element of fertility treatment. The correlation between the scale of oocyte procurement and successful conception comes as something of a shock to women in IVF treatment, and the valuation of oocytes emerges directly from the dawning realization that their hopes for a child revolve around this correlation. Women in IVF come to regard their oocytes as "precious," indeed as "beyond price," and they become deeply invested in maximizing the opportunity for the fertilization of each egg. At the same time, this correlation produces the steep demand for third-party oocytes, either through donation proper or through various kinds of transaction. To put it another way, IVF is the necessary condition for an oocyte economy proper to emerge, and I explore the conditions for this economy in this chapter.

In what follows, I draw on interviews carried out between 2009 and 2011 with three groups: twenty women who were ex-IVF patients, five women who had donated oocytes to other women for reproductive purposes, and ten clinicians who worked with these women as nursing, counseling, and scientific staff. The study, which focused on donation decisions for stem cell research, used in-depth qualitative interviews to establish the complexity of such decisions. The women were recruited through a large fertility clinic in Sydney. Of the twenty IVF patients and five reproductive donors, all except one were married or in a de facto relationship, and thirteen had a university-level education. All identified as heterosexual. Eight IVF participants did not have a live birth from their treatment. Of these, seven stated that they would continue with IVF in the future. Five IVF patients were aged over forty years at the time of the interview, and three participants had an oocyte or embryo donor.

IVF
Hope and Uncertainty

In vitro fertilization, and the broader set of practices termed "assisted reproductive technology" (ART), has become a relatively common experience. The treatment type I most concerned about in this study is IVF, but other types of ART include intrauterine insemination, donor insemination, intracytoplasmic sperm injection (ICSI), and preimplantation genetic diagnosis (PGD). Recent estimates of the global figures for reproductive treatment indicate that for the years 2008, 2009, and 2010, 4,461,309 ART cycles were initiated, and an estimated 1,144,858 babies were born as a result (Dyer et al. 2016). Despite this routinization, IVF retains some of the features of its earlier experimental status. In particular, the process is highly uncertain. While the success rate for IVF has increased incrementally since the 1980s, the most probable outcome for any treatment cycle is failure. Longitudinal data from Australia and New Zealand, following women through treatment over time, found that the live delivery rate for each treatment cycle was 14.0–17.0 percent. If these ratios are segmented by age, live delivery rates for women aged under thirty was 26.0 percent, while for those over forty-four, the live delivery rate was 0.9 percent (Macaldowie et al. 2014). UK statistics indicate a similar distribution of live births per treatment: 32.2 percent for women under thirty-five, 27.7 percent for women aged thirty-five to thirty-seven, 20.8 percent for women aged thirty-eight to thirty-nine, 13.6 percent for women aged forty to forty-two, 5.0 percent for women aged forty-three to forty-four, and 1.9 percent for women over forty-four (National Health Service 2013). The same picture emerges from U.S. data, with 40.5 percent of women under thirty-five having a live birth, but only 1.8 percent of women over forty-four (National Center for Chronic Disease Prevention and Health Promotion 2014).

Reputable fertility clinics present these somewhat daunting statistics to women seeking treatment. Yet women entering into IVF tend toward optimism about their chances of a happy outcome. The reasons for this overestimation are complex, but among the participants in this study, we can discern a general overestimation of the technical capabilities of the fertility clinic. Women and couples do not generally turn to IVF without at least a year of failed attempts at unassisted conception, and they may have endured miscarriage, ectopic pregnancies, and other kinds of distressing experiences (Miller 2007; Mahon 2014). When they present for treatment, they are likely to hope that, given they have a *mechanical* problem with their reproductive biology, there must also be a *mechanical* solution, a technical fix. This hope is both fostered and quelled by clinics; fostered through marketing images of beautiful, smiling infants and success rates compared to competitors, and quelled when potential patients are presented with their generally low chances of conception per cycle.

Among the women interviewed, many began treatment quite confident that they would conceive in their first cycle and were surprised to find themselves among the statistical majority, without a child (Carroll and Waldby 2012). As Mandy put it,

> I really—I looked at the statistics and everything, so I didn't go in blind, but I thought, "Oh, I'll be one of the, whatever it was, twenty something percent: no, I'll be one of those." And the people it doesn't work for, well they must have other, there must be other serious issues for them. But that's not necessarily the case: there's lots of people that go through without success and it's not necessarily explained, but . . . I just think that it will work (slight laugh); we'll just keep trying, and we've made so many changes to our lives and there's nothing else that we could possible do, really." (Mandy, ex-IVF patient, mid-thirties, nurse, married, no children)

Karen Throsby, in her study of the experience of IVF failure, notes that her participants tended to foreground the "naturalness" of IVF, as a technical assistant to their own natural reproductive potential, while also, paradoxically, considering it to be high-technology medicine, an element of modern technical progress. "A distinction between *helping* nature and *tampering* with nature is crucial to the construction of IVF as fundamentally natural, and ultimately, uncomplicated, both morally and technologically. From this perspective, IVF becomes not only analogous to the natural, but is itself rendered within the natural domain" (Throsby 2004, 61). Sarah Franklin observes moreover that the naturalness of IVF is *intrinsic* to its technical and biological design. "It replicates a well-known biological process, namely fertilization, and confirms the ability to simulate this process technologically. . . . Representations of IVF typically reproduce, and condense, familiar narratives—from the naturalness of reproduction and the universal desire for parenthood to the value of scientific progress and the benefits of medical assistance" (Franklin 2013, 6). The point in these two analyses is that, irrespective of the scientific claims or marketing strategies of particular clinics, the historical propagation of IVF technologies has inflected it with a naturalized ethos, a sense that the technical interventions simply augment biological processes.

This optimistic interpretation of IVF as a linear, technical enhancement, something that can be added to one's slightly deficient reproductive biology to reliably produce a child, is somewhat perturbed by the experience of being in actual treatment. Only once the women interviewed had been through at least one entire cycle of treatment did they fully appreciated the nonlinear, nonadditive nature of IVF, and the highly unpredictable interaction between technical procedures and their own or their partner's biology. As one Australian fertility nurse noted, this realization can sometimes be expressed as anger toward the clinic and the fertility specialists:

> [The patients ask,] "Why can't you just fix it for me? I'm coming to you; I'm giving you my time, I'm doing what you're telling me and you're the expert—why isn't it working?" And unfortunately we don't have those answers, so. . . . But yeah, their expectation is like, "I'll do everything you tell me!" It's like the bank, you know, or like a transaction or like a contract: "I'll fulfill my side of the bargain and then what I'm asking for you is to make me pregnant. And [I'm] not, so what happened?"

Above all, after one treatment cycle, women discover the extent to which the chances of successful conception, pregnancy, and birth pivot on the number and quality of oocytes that can be procured as the first step in treatment.

The Deficit Spiral

The techniques of IVF create the preconditions for the development of an oocyte economy in two senses. First, they make oocytes into potentially *transactable* objects. Second, they create oocyte *deficits*. Without IVF, oocytes remain singular and in vivo, inaccessible to technical or social circulation. Most women, in the course of their menstrual cycle, will produce one mature oocyte each month, which remains in the body and, if not fertilized, will be lost during menstruation. As we saw in the previous chapter, the development of techniques to produce viable ex vivo human oocytes took almost a century of tinkering with mammalian reproductive biology, and contemporary IVF treatment is a clinical refinement of this experimental history.

In vitro fertilization is only possible if both sets of gametes, eggs and sperm, can be manipulated under laboratory conditions. While this is relatively straightforward for sperm procurement, grafting itself onto the biology of ejaculation, it is not at all straightforward for oocytes. Charis Thompson coins the term "ontological choreography" to designate the daunting complexity of the clinical social and legal processes that must be coordinated for an IVF treatment to take place. "Ontological choreography," she writes,

> refers to the dynamic coordination of the technical, scientific, kinship, gender, emotional, legal, political, and financial aspects of ART clinics. What might appear to be an undifferentiated hybrid mess is actually a deftly balanced coming together of things that are generally considered parts of different ontological orders (part of nature, part of the self, part of society). These elements have to be coordinated in highly staged ways so as to get on with the task at hand: producing parents, children, and everything that is needed for their recognition as such. Thus, for example, at specific moments a body part and surgical instruments must stand in a specific relationship, at other times a legal decision can disambiguate kinship in countless subsequent procedures, and at other times a bureaucratic accounting form can protect the sanctity of the human embryo or allow certain embryos to be discarded. Although this kind of choreography between different kinds of things goes on to some extent in all spheres of human activity, it is especially striking in ART clinics. (Thompson 2005, 8)

While Thompson is concerned with an inclusive account of the entire assisted reproductive experience, her point regarding the highly staged coordination of disparate elements is apt when we focus on the more specific dimension of oocyte procurement. The first and most physically onerous part of IVF treatment for women is the process of ovarian stimulation and egg retrieval, to scale up and externalize oocyte production so that the cells can be fertilized in the laboratory.

During ovarian stimulation the woman subscribes to a complex daily hormonal drug regime. At the outset, ovarian activity is suppressed, using a nasal spray for approximately two weeks to induce what is effectively a brief menopause. The next stage involves a daily or sometimes twice daily administration of follicle-stimulating hormone (FSH) to stimulate the production and maturation of multiple oocytes in the ovaries. The hormone is administered by subcutaneous injection, and this is usually undertaken by the woman herself, rather than in a clinic. While some women find this aspect unproblematic, several interviewees reported considerable anxiety about using the syringe, at least initially:

I had the alarm set for one injection in the morning and one at night; the alarm goes off and that's the alarm to get up in the morning, you know? It gets a bit overwhelming. As I said, it's a means to an end, so for me, it's just something that I have to go through. . . . I've never had to inject myself, so getting used to all that was a little bit daunting; making sure you're doing it correctly and what have you. (Dominique, ex-IVF patient, mid-thirties, chef, de facto relationship, no children)

The injections must be made at the same time each day, and they put something of a strain on women with work and family schedules. They also involve the management of awkward and potentially embarrassing drug paraphernalia. In Throsby's study, women describe juggling syringes in their workplace toilets and carrying handbags full of complicated, time-critical medications that they must take while in the middle of a meeting or traveling on the London Underground (Throsby 2002). The rate of oocyte production is monitored through transvaginal ultrasound and blood tests, so women have to visit to the clinic for regular examinations. One interviewee describes the difficulties of regular, timed self-administration and clinic attendance while caring for small children:

I guess because, having the boys . . . there was no need for them to know about it, and I think it's a bit complicated for them to [have it] explained anyway, and having to have the injections at a certain time every day. . . . A couple of times we were away and I had to . . . take [the medication] with me and do it wherever I was, so I guess, yeah, just trying to stick to that routine with all the other demands of children and so on was a bit challenging. (Serena, reproductive donor, mid-thirties, married, student, two children)

There is no simple, linear relationship between the dosage levels of FSH and the number of oocytes collected, although higher dosages tend to produce more oocytes. The interviewees indicated that large numbers of oocytes in the ovaries were associated with more discomfort, pain, and bloating than smaller numbers.

It was my first [treatment], I was feeling really kind of nauseous and . . . you know, I was finding it difficult walking, like I almost walked with a limp because it was so painful; you know, I'd go in the car, and every little bump, I felt like I had lead weights holding my ovaries down, so every little bump, I could feel it and I'd be like, "Oh *gosh!*" Like yeah, because [my ovaries] were just *huge*. . . . I think the first time, you're blinded to what IVF can be [like]. (Mira, ex-IVF patient, early thirties, married, home worker, one child)

The women also described the hormone-enhanced mood swings, made more acute by their intense hopes and fears about their chances of conception. These hopes and fears, the anxieties and desire for mother-hood, play a decisive part here, as Rene Almeling and Iris Willey's recent study demonstrates. Comparing the accounts of paid oocyte donors with those of women undergoing IVF to conceive their own child, they found a wide disparity. "Women doing in vitro fertilization (IVF) to have a child describe it as painful and emotionally draining. Egg donors undergo the same medical regimen for a different reason: to produce eggs for another woman in exchange for thousands of dollars and describe it as quick and relatively painless" (Almeling and Willey 2017, 21). We can see here the *ontological dimensions* of Thompson's ontological choreography, the extent to which oocyte procurement, and IVF more generally, interweaves the technical with the personal and with the structure of feeling around maternal identification and desire.

Sarah gives an eloquent account of these dynamics. She states that the first treatment cycle was the most precipitous, in the sense that her expectations had not yet been tempered by the experience of repeated failure:

The first time around, it was exciting but anxious and then disappoint-ing with the outcome. The second time around, it was like riding a bike and from there on in it is very straightforward. . . . But yeah, it's probably more a case of being aware of the intense hormonal influ-ences on your body. And the mood swings and things that actually occur; you have *extremes* of emotion but it's probably the same as pregnancy, where you get extremely happy or extremely depressed or extremely angry and you go through all these extremes while you're under the influence of the hormone medication. (Sarah, ex-IVF pa-tient, late thirties, accountant, married, one child)

About two weeks after initiating the injections, if the oocytes are suf-ficiently developed, the patients are administered a trigger injection, which signals the ovaries to release the oocytes. Collection takes place thirty-six hours later, in day surgery, under sedation, using a transvaginal procedure. Precise timing is crucial at this point, because if collection takes place too soon, the oocytes may not be sufficiently mature. Once collected, they are treated for several hours to optimize maturation and then fertilized with the partner's or donor semen. Clinic staff will usually attempt to fertilize all the mature oocytes retrieved. For the women interviewed, this point in the process involves the most anxiety and potential disappointment. The IVF patient must wait between two and five days to see if a viable blastocyst (early embryo) develops from the process. No successful fertilization may result, and the entire process may be for naught. They must then decide whether to undergo another cycle. Most of the women reported being excited and hopeful with their first procedure, but their optimism deflated as the reality of failed cycles came home:

> I think [for] your first cycle, you're kind of excited, and I remember saying to someone, "This isn't as hard as what everyone supposedly reckons it is. I've heard IVF is really hard. It's not that hard." And the first time, it's quite exciting, and if that doesn't work you get to the second time and you're all excited and gee'd up and that doesn't work and then, you know. (Caroline, ex-IVF patient, early thirties, sales manager, married, no children)

So, in summary, oocyte stimulation is a very prolonged and invasive process, and almost all the women described it as onerous. In addition to the evident physical demands, women who have generally tried for years to conceive experience the stress associated with the sense that this is their last chance to have a child, so that each step in the process is burdened with anxiety and expectation. In short, the production of ex vivo oocytes requires considerable commitment, effort, endurance, and courage, and women's valuation of their oocytes are shaped by these demands.

The technology of IVF is organized around the production of multiple oocytes, the creation of abundance. I would argue, however, somewhat counterintuitively, that fertility treatment produces structural oocyte *deficits*, which are intrinsic to the system of IVF. These deficits set the conditions through which women come to think of their own eggs as precious, to be safeguarded and protected. They also set the conditions for the global oocyte *market*, creating a demand for oocytes provided by other women, generally for money, if patients find that they cannot produce their own. To understand this systematic deficit, we need to consider more closely the ways in which the techniques of IVF lack certain kinds of traction over the material qualities of oocytes.

As reproductive tissues pass through the various stages in the IVF process, they are subject to something of a negative cascade, or deficit spiral. Each step in the process successively blocks off options and pathways, so that the odds mount against successful reproduction at each point: in vivo eggs need to become mature in vitro eggs, which in turn need to successfully fertilize with sperm in vitro. The sperm needs to be motile and fertile, qualities not necessarily easy to determine. If sperm is of poor quality, an ICSI may be necessary, or the couple may need to find donor sperm.[2] The fertilized eggs need to become blastocysts, which are graded for their viability in terms of cell quantity, quality and arrangement, and the expansion of the embryo. In vitro embryos need to develop sufficiently to become transferable embryos, which are then either placed in the woman's uterus or frozen for later use. Frozen embryos need to survive the thaw, to return to the status of transferable embryos. Transferable embryos then need to become secure pregnancies that, in turn, are carried to term and result in a live birth.

At each of these points, the process may go wrong, and the odds at any given point are in part determined by the number and quality of reproductive units (oocytes, sperm, fresh embryos, frozen embryos) available at the previous stage. Moreover, women treated through IVF have slightly higher odds of miscarriage, so that even if they establish an apparently viable pregnancy, they are less likely to go to term and give birth (Herbert, Lucke, and Dobson 2009; Gunby et al. 2010).

Eva's experience succinctly encapsulates both the difficulties of repeated cycles and the deficit spiral that leads downward from a sometimes high number of oocytes to miscarriage and disappointment.

I think they collected less than ten, because the first, with my daughter—I remember there was, like, sixteen. There was a lot. So this was, maybe, six eggs. I think we got five embryos out of that. One was transferred. There must have been four embryos. One was transferred and three were frozen. So, the fresh cycle didn't work. Tried a frozen one, didn't work. Went to try the third frozen and they told me that one didn't survive unfreezing, so then we had one left and that didn't work, so we had no embryos left. So we did a fresh cycle again, and they got even less this time. I remember them saying that the sperm were immature, so I was thinking that—like, the day that they did the embryo—because when they collect my eggs is when they do the ICSI, take the sperm out, so they do it at the same time. I remember my husband coming back and saying that they look immature, so I was thinking this is all going to be wasting time, but they got—I think they fertilized four eggs, and then there was only one viable one, which is this baby. (Eva, ex-IVF patient, early thirties, teacher, married, one child)

Oocytes constitute the most fragile and least tractable point in the woman's reproductive process. Even if treatment produces a large number of oocytes, their viability is not guaranteed. Moreover, treatment may produce a small number of viable oocytes in one cycle, while another cycle may produce a large number of unviable ones. Oocytes are initially graded for their degree of maturity, but this is not a measure of fertility per se. No validated laboratory test, at time of writing, can tell clinicians which ones to use and which ones to discard. While proposals are in circulation in the field regarding ways to grade oocytes (e.g., Lazzaroni-Tealdi et al. 2015), there is no clinical consensus. In practice, the way to tell if an oocyte is fertile is to fertilize it.

Moreover, while blastocysts are routinely banked for future conception attempts, oocytes are not routinely frozen. While some clinics now use cryopreservation for oocytes, this is not yet standard practice, and most clinics still prefer to fertilize all eggs when they are fresh. (I investigate the new terrain of egg freezing in chapters 5 and 6.)

Because of these dwindling odds, IVF patients are forced to engage in what Erica Haimes and Ken Taylor term the "calculus of conception," a drawn-out negotiation with the clinicians about how best to maximize the particular combination of reproductive materials they have at their disposal: "We use this phrase to convey the mental arithmetic that patients endlessly perform to calculate their chances of achieving a baby from the number of follicles, eggs, fertilised eggs, cells and embryos they have succeeded in producing. The calculations gain complexity by considerations of quality ['it's drummed into you, it's quality, not quantity that counts' (IVF40:833–852)] and by the choices between different uses of these entities" (Haimes and Taylor 2009, 2144).

Oocytes are the tissues that sit at the top of this stream of decisions and calculations, but I would argue that they also sit outside it. Of all the reproductive tissues and technical decision points involved in IVF, they are the material least open to quantification and instrumental reasoning, because of their stochastic, nonlinear biological properties and the imprecision of the effects generated by hormonal treatment. As tissues, oocytes could be said to lack predictable input-output ratios: no precise relationship exists between amounts of hormone stimulation and numbers produced, nor do high numbers imply high fertility odds, because most may be unviable. In this sense, they sit outside the IVF patient's "calculus of conception," while forming the conditions of its possibility. Oocytes are themselves inscrutable and incalculable, but they set the parameters for calculation further downstream.

Incalculable Potential

These opaque qualities and their position at the top of the process are the conditions that set the inestimable value of oocytes for the women going through IVF. I use the term "inestimable" to indicate both their precious quality, the sense that each egg has a high degree of personal worth derived from the effort to produce them, and their incalculable quality, their resistance to ranking, division, and hierarchy. These qualities are closely linked. For women in treatment, and indeed for clinicians and embryologists, there is no agreed method of estimating the *comparative value* of each egg (Rienzi et al. 2011). The only reliable test for each oocyte's fertility is to fertilize it, so that its fertile potential is proved at the same time it is spent. In this sense, each unfertilized oocyte has an equal degree of preciousness because each has an *incalculable potential*. Each represents the same unknowable chance for the desired child, and each degree of potential can only be known retrospectively, after the attempt.

The women repeatedly described the experience of producing quite high number of eggs, only to find that most failed to fertilize. Francesca describes this precipitous drop from apparent potential to unrealized hope.

> We had fifteen eggs. Out of ten, only one was fertile; it became an embryo. Obviously we had that one implanted. I then became pregnant and miscarried ten weeks later, so that was quite devastating. I had to go through the whole process *again*. The second time I had thirty

eggs taken out, which was *very* painful. Out of thirty . . . we had eight successful. One was implanted, which was successful and went full-term, thirty-nine weeks, with the pregnancy. We got seven embryos frozen. (Francesca, ex-IVF patient, late twenties, travel consultant, married, one child)

Francesca's experience nicely demonstrates the incalculability of oocytes, the apparently random allocation of fertile capacity across each egg in a cycle, the mercurial fluctuation of fertility between cycles, the dilation and extinction of hope, as their potential proves elusive and illusory.

This opaque potential was expressed by the women and some of the clinicians in relation to the "one" egg needed for a successful pregnancy, irrespective of the number of eggs actually produced through stimulation. As one fertility nurse put it,

> Yes, they need one egg, but how do you . . . choose what that one egg is? How do you know which is the egg that's going to make it?

Each egg has the same incalculable value, and each egg is invested with the same degree of hope. This found its most acute expression in the almost complete unwillingness of women to consider donating oocytes produced during treatment. In Joanna's words,

> [I couldn't donate] during [IVF], because then I'd be thinking, "Oh, that might have been the good egg that could have got me pregnant!" So no, I couldn't. (Joanna, ex-IVF patient, late twenties, insurance agent, married, no children)

Joanna is acutely aware that diverting even one oocyte to research, or to reproductive donation, could involve the diminution of her entire fertility potential, because there is no way to estimate the distribution of fertility among a cycle of oocytes. Oocytes do not constitute equal, divisible units of reproductive potential, where rational decisions can be made to allocate a proportion to research or to another woman and keep a proportion for oneself. Our respondents were confronted with the possibility that they might give away their most (or only) fertile oocyte without knowing it and find themselves bereft. As Isabel puts it:

> I guess the reason why I'm going through the treatment is to fall pregnant, so I want the best option I've got to fall pregnant, and that means getting the most out of the eggs that they've taken from me to increase

my chances of falling pregnant. I understand there are other people who've got fertility issues as well, and some people that IVF doesn't work for, so they need people to donate so they can actually understand why they can't fall pregnant, but they're getting extremely selfish. It's a really big thing to go through IVF, and I'm doing it for myself. Again, it took us so long to decide to go through it in the first place, so I don't want to diminish my chances of falling pregnant by giving away the only viable egg out of everything that they've taken from me. You're not going to know until they fertilize them. (Isabel, ex-IVF patient, late thirties, married, one child, marketing professional)

Of the twenty ex-patient women interviewed, only four would contemplate donating their eggs to medical research during their own treatment, and only those eggs that failed to fertilize. A slightly greater proportion would consider reproductive donation, but only under highly specific conditions. They typically stated things like,

If it was . . . a loved one that desperately wanted a child, then yes. Other than that, I would struggle to do that [egg collection] again. (Francesca, ex-IVF patient, late twenties, travel consultant, married, one child)

The incalculable qualities of oocytes are thrown into relief when we compare the interviewees' attitudes toward the donation of embryos. While they were extremely unwilling to contemplate egg donation, all stated that they would be prepared to donate embryos for medical research. The women stated in different ways that they did not want to *waste* embryos. Bridget's response is typical:

Because it's such a waste, isn't it? They just sort of get put down the gurgler and nothing gets done with them. (Bridget, ex-IVF patient, early forties, shop assistant, married, one child, pregnant with second)

This preparedness to donate to another arises because IVF embryos differ from IVF eggs in two principle biotechnical ways: first, they can be ranked, and second, they can be stored. Clinicians grade blastocysts according to a range of morphological and chromosomal biomarkers. They will discard those that are unlikely to develop and pick the most viable-looking blastocyst for transfer to the woman's uterus, while others will be frozen for use if the first fails. Among the respondents, approximately one-third had embryos in storage. Bridget's reference to the embryos being "put down the gurgler" describes the process of disposal for these embryos. Once a couple decides they no longer need them, frozen embryos are disposed of through the clinic's biological waste management process, unless they are donated.[3]

These are decisive qualities. Ranking means that the woman or couple has a *quantified* sense of the blastocyst's potential for development, and a way to compare one with another. While, like oocytes, blastocysts are invested with a great deal of hope, they are less prone to inexplicable reversals because they are less opaque. They are also a *divisible* resource. Because only viable embryos are banked, each embryo represents a roughly equivalent unit of potential, so that rational decisions can be made about their division and allocation. Oocytes cannot be rationally divided in this way because of their mercurial distributions of fertility.

At the same time, cryopreservation creates a margin of deliberation for women or couples wishing to consider the best way to deploy their embryos. Freezing removes embryos from time-critical processes to some extent. It creates a pause in the relentless choreography of conception and gives couples the ability to defer decisions about them until after completing treatment. Hence, frozen embryos can be designated as *surplus* once couples reach a certain point in the IVF trajectory and given to another without endangering their reproductive hopes. In summary, the reproductive value of embryos can be both apportioned and deferred, while that of oocytes cannot. *For IVF patients, the reproductive value of oocytes must be spent in the present, and spent all at once.* This calculus may be changing, at least for younger women (those under thirty-five), as oocyte cryopreservation techniques improve, and some clinics move toward routine oocyte banking as part of their suite of services to clients, a change discussed at length in chapters 5 and 6.

Deficit and Donation

In this fashion, material constraints on oocyte production and viability create fertility deficits for women going through IVF. They struggle to produce sufficient fertile eggs to create a viable pregnancy, and may embark on cycle after cycle, as even generous numbers fail to create grade one blastocysts, and a failed cycle may presage a more successful one. Women in treatment are, for these reasons, extremely unwilling to donate eggs to other women. Consequently, there is no ready way to increase the supply of allogeneic fertility without soliciting donation from women who are not themselves in need of fertility treatment. The act of donation involves the same hormonal stimulation process as IVF: multiple medications, clinic visits, and extended, committed kinds of compliance that interfere with the demands of work and family. It lacks the aura of therapeutic public good that accrues to blood and solid organ donation, with their promise of life-saving action (Healy 2006). In summary, it involves a much greater burden or risk, time, and discomfort for the donor while lacking the heroic narrative associated with therapeutic donation. The net effect of this configuration is that few women consent to donate eggs in the *strict* sense of the gift relation as it is articulated in the foundational, twentieth-century arguments (Jonas 1969; Titmuss [1970] 1997), as a moral obligation to contribute freely to the public good, without incentive or transaction (Waldby and Mitchell 2006).

This unwillingness is evident in the comparatively low numbers of donor-assisted treatment cycles in jurisdictions that enforce strict gifting for oocytes. In Ireland, for example, where donation is governed by strict Irish Medical Council gifting guidelines, only twenty egg donation cycles were reported from seven clinics and 4,078 treatment cycles (0.5 percent) in 2010. In the same year Spain, which permits high rates of cash-based compensation, reports 12,928 donation cycles from 58,735 treatments (22.0 percent) (Kupka et al. 2014). In Victoria, Australia, 369 women received donor oocytes during 2013–14, from a total of 10,598 women in fertility treatment (roughly 3.5 percent; Victorian Assisted Reproductive Treatment Authority 2014). In Australia and New Zealand as a whole, oocyte donor cycles represented 2.7 percent of all treatment cycles in 2013, and the average age of women receiving donation was 40.7 (Macaldowie et al. 2015). These Australian figures reflect the continued national commitment to regulating oocyte donation as a gift relation. Under section 21 of the Prohibition of Human Cloning and the Regulation of Human Embryo Research Amendment Act 2006, the exchange of oocytes for money is illegal and punishable by fifteen years' imprisonment, but "donors may be compensated for any reasonable expenses incurred relating to collection, storage or transport of donated oöcytes or sperm." Such expenses may include those associated with attending appointments, and reimbursement for associated costs of childcare, transport, and the like. Donors cannot be offered inducement, nor can they profit from donation.

In Australia, the term "compensation" is generally interpreted narrowly, to mean the reimbursement of documented costs, while in Spain, a high-donation country, compensation is interpreted liberally. I discuss some of the consequences of this difference in chapter 4, "Global Oocytes."

Hence, oocyte donors in Australia demonstrate considerable altruism, and in what follows, I want to consider this group in a little more detail. Here I am particularly interested in how they understand their contribution to their recipient's child, and the circumstances that led them to understand their eggs as surplus, an excess that they can afford to give, rather than as precious and scarce.

Altruistic Donation

A small number of empirical studies investigate altruistic oocyte donation. Louise Byrd, Mary Sidebotham, and Brian Lieberman (2002) surveyed 113 reproductive egg donors in the UK and found that their overwhelming motivation to donate was a desire to help childless couples. A large survey-based study carried out by Guido Pennings and colleagues found that of 1,423 egg donors located in eleven European countries (Belgium, Czech Republic, Finland, France, Greece, Poland, Portugal, Russia, Spain, Ukraine, and the UK), almost 50 percent of the sample stated that their motivation to donate was purely altruistic and based on a desire to help others have a family (Pennings et al. 2014). Altruistic donors were more likely to be older (above thirty-five years), well educated, citizens of the country where the clinic was located, and working full time. These kinds of donations were more evident in jurisdictions with low levels of compensation or with strict reimbursement (e.g., France) and were more likely to be first time donors, while women who reported a strictly financial motivation (10.8 percent of respondents) were more likely to be repeat donors, to be students or working part time, and to receive high rates of compensation (Greece, Russia). Pennings and colleagues (2014) note that the country with the strictest regulations around reimbursement produced the highest percentage of altruistic donors, but a low number of donors overall. This is broadly consonant with the situation in Australia.

In my study, we interviewed five women who had donated to another in Sydney, Australia, and found a similar concern to aid childless couples and help create a happy family (Boulos 2014; Boulos, Kerridge, and Waldby 2014). While egg donation is not, strictly speaking, therapeutic, the donors nevertheless clearly regarded childlessness as a form of suffering and considered that they had the means to alleviate that suffering through their generosity. In four of the five cases, they did not know the couple personally, but rather responded to a plea published in local media.

I remember just feeling very intensely that if I could help them, I would like to, because it's something that she wanted so much. . . . I just thought [to] myself how awful it would be, having had two children, to feel that I couldn't have fulfilled being a parent. (Serena, reproductive donor, late thirties, married, student, two children)

[I saw an ad] In the *Wentworth Courier*! They'd been married for a long time, been trying for eleven years, and I've always thought about doing it. I don't want children of my own, and so I thought if I could help someone else to do it. . . . They're a really nice couple. We met a few times over coffee. I met the wife first, and then I met the husband, and they're just a really nice couple. Yeah. So that's why I only did it for them, not . . . yeah. (Christine, reproductive donor, early thirties, nurse, engaged, no children)

Egg donation under Australian conditions tends to be quite a personal process, because, as a rule, clinics do not broker donation, and couples are advised that they will need to identify a donor themselves. They generally seek donors through print advertisements and can only hope for a respondent. Agnes, one of the donors interviewed, describes her surprise on finding a long list of advertisements pleading for a donor in the back of a magazine.

To me, more than anything . . . me personally, I think there would be nothing worse than not being able to have children. . . . And it happened that just spontaneously during the day I was reading a children's magazine and flipped the page and saw an ad for an egg donor, and then when I took a step back I saw that there was, like, an A3 page worth of women with advertisements just asking for egg donors, and that sort of got me thinking, going, "What's going on?" So I went and did the research, and didn't actually realize how prevalent it was, and how common it was, that women couldn't. (Agnes, reproductive donor, late twenties, teacher, de facto relationship, no children)

So unlike therapeutic donation, where blood and organs are given anonymously, through systems that carefully ensure a lack of knowledge and contact (Mamode et al. 2013), egg donation in Australia depends on donor and recipient identifying and negotiating with each other, often over protracted periods. Donors talked about the importance for them of the personal nature of these bonds, the sense that they were giving not to an anonymous third party but to a specific couple, with whom they had sympathy.

> I guess having known them and spoken to them and really kind of connected with their emotional needs and wants to have a child and so on, I could really kind of relate to that . . . yeah. So maybe it was just having that personal connection that made me feel like I wanted to do it. (Serena, reproductive donor, late thirties, married, student, two children)

The five donors interviewed were prepared to consider donation because they felt that they did not need their own eggs, or they did not need them any longer. Either they had completed their families (in three cases) and felt compassion for women unable to do so, or they felt strongly that they did not want children themselves (in two cases). As Meg, mother of one child and pregnant with another, put it,

> No—I gave them a little bit of space at the beginning, because I think I just had to get my head around it; but the fact that I'm pregnant now too kind of makes me feel a little bit better about it, because I'll have my own baby. And I've already got my own—I don't think I would've donated it, if I didn't have my own child in the first place. (Meg, reproductive donor, early thirties, teacher, married, one child and pregnant with second)

So these women could donate to another either because the potential of their eggs had already been satisfactorily realized with the creation of their own children, or because they did not plan to realize that potential in the *capacity of mother*. Rather, they were happy to give that potential away, to be realized elsewhere by others. This did not mean, however, that they were disinterested in the outcome of the treatment cycle. All five donors explained that they had assessed their recipient couple as good parents and considered that they had a responsibility to any child born through the process to ensure that they were born into a good home.

Meg explained further, "Um, I think because they were so great to kids anyway. And I know they'd been trying—they were so good to my first, my Patrick, my son; and I thought, 'God! You'd make great parents.' And they're just so caring, and they give to everybody else—I was like, 'Oh well, it's time that you got something back'" (Meg, reproductive donor, early thirties, teacher, married, one child and pregnant with second). Agnes expressed similar feelings: "I did want to meet them. I want to, sort of, know that my eggs are going at least to someone who's worthy of them, in a sense. I don't know if that sounds bad or not . . . yeah. I think maybe if I didn't feel right about the thing, maybe I would have pulled out" (Agnes, reproductive donor, late twenties, teacher, de facto relationship, no children).

Donors were also invested in the practical success of the treatment cycle. Three of the five first cycles failed to produce a pregnancy, and donors reported their feelings of disappointment and dismay:

> From what they were able to [tell] me, they actually didn't get a lot of success from that . . . I thought, a couple [of embryos] died, then when you freeze them, then they defrost, a few more die. So they tried once or twice, and it was unsuccessful. And then they had like two left in the freezer, so to speak, and I said, "Oh, because you haven't really had much of a go, how about we have *another* go of it?" So I donated again—that was the beginning of this year, and I donated again, and they got another seven eggs. So from that exact transfer, she fell pregnant! (Meg, reproductive donor, early thirties, teacher, married, one child and pregnant with second)

As I argue elsewhere, women tend to feel a profound sense of responsibility about reproductive donation, both for oocytes and embryos, in the sense that they want to be sure that the life they help create will be born into a caring family. This concern is often the reason women and couples are disinclined to donate their spare embryos anonymously to other couples and prefer research donation, as they fear the possibility of abuse or neglect (Cooper and Waldby 2014). This concern for the welfare of the child is evident among the group of interviewees. Hence their interest in vetting the intending parents. In one case, this concern extended to a continuing relationship with the intending parents and inclusion in the child's care. For the most part, however, donors were careful to distance themselves from the status of mother, and to explicitly constitute their donation as a pragmatic, instrumental kind of assistance (Boulos 2014). As Meg states, she is already a mother and does not need the status of mother to donor-conceived offspring.

> At the end of the day, it's just an egg. If I didn't have my own children and I'd donated, I actually don't think you'd be able to disconnect so much. Because I think you'd go, "Well, I don't have any children, and you've got that one, which I helped you with." So having my own children means, "You know what? I've got my own—I don't need. . . ." So that's not a worry for me as much anymore.

She continues, explaining her emotional difficulties in making such a clear separation between herself and the resulting child:

> It's been a little up and down—I can get a little emotional at times. . . . Your brain still has to disconnect from the fact that it's got nothing to do with you, even though this child is going to look like you and have your same mannerisms, it's not yours. . . . And seeing her pregnant. . . . It's actually very good, because you know, as soon as you see someone pregnant—"That's not your kid; that's theirs." (Meg, reproductive donor, early thirties, teacher, married, one child and pregnant with second)

Here we can see Meg engage in a delicate rationalization about the status of her donated oocytes. She constitutes the egg recipient as the mother because the recipient gestates the child to term and will give birth to and raise it. In this respect she is grappling with how assisted reproductive technologies *redistribute* maternity, so that the biology of ovulation, conception, gestation, and birth can be disaggregated from one another and apportioned to two or three different women.

Conclusion

The redistribution of fertility and the allocation of partial biological motherhood to several different women in the creation of one child is perhaps the most profound social complication of ARTS. It unsettles historical understandings of maternal claim as a singular status, where biology and legal qualities are made coterminous. Note, however, that there are significant historical exceptions to this unification of biological and legal claims. Forced appropriation of children from their unmarried biological mothers and reallocation to more respectable families form an important part of the history of twentieth-century reproduction (Zamostny et al. 2003), and the earlier history of slavery in the United States and Europe saw routine appropriation of children from mothers who lacked any civil status (Beckles 1989). Family structures in nineteenth-century Australia and Britain also routinely distributed some of the facets of maternity that would seem more properly unified to contemporary sensibilities, particularly contracting wet nurses for breastfeeding (Waldby 1983).

So when we consider how assisted reproduction redistributes maternity, we should treat the norm of legal and biological unification as already historically contingent. Nevertheless, in Meg's account above, and in much of the discussion of women's experiences of donor-assisted conception and egg freezing in the remainder of the book, this dynamic presents particularly poignant difficulties of feeling and identification. Clinics, policy makers, and regulators invest considerable effort in managing this aspect of ARTS. Indeed, for Charis Thompson, the disambiguation of conflicting maternal claims and statuses is a particularly difficult element in the ontological choreography performed by the clinic, as assisted reproduction disaggregates the properties of motherhood *in new ways* (Thompson 2005). The most entrenched ethical scandals around ARTS relate to the contestation of claims to primary motherhood, particularly those created by gestational surrogacy (Schover 2014; Whittaker 2016).

In Australia, the birth mother is the legal mother in family law, and Meg's comments, and indeed the entire practice of egg donation, rest on this understanding.[4] At the same time, however, Meg is engaged in a rationalization about the capacities and status of her oocytes; in saying "it's just an egg," she is foregrounding the instrumental capacities of the oocyte, its biological action in conception, embryogenesis, and the establishment of gestation. It is the cell necessary for the creation of the embryo and the pregnancy, but the actual gestation, birth, and nurturing constitute the *maternal relation* in her reasoning (Boulos 2014). To rationalize along these lines, however, she necessarily reduces the ontological and generational capacities of her oocytes, their ability to transmit her specific genetic identity and that of her antecedents. In short, she discounts the significance of these capacities in the duration of fertility and the transmission of generational time for the purposes of donation. She already has children, so she has already realized this ontological and

generational potential and feels she can regard her eggs in a more instrumental and disinterested light.

Nevertheless, she struggles to make a clean separation between these
various qualities and can't perfectly detach herself from a sense of care,
obligation, and vigilance regarding the welfare and status of the child. As
I discuss in the next chapter, the *recipients* of oocyte donation struggle in
a similar fashion to feel entitled to the child. While oocytes have a highly
pragmatic, instrumental value, as the means to the desired child, they are
inescapably invested with personal and family significance and complex
maternal claims. The redistribution of maternal capacities effected by IVF
necessarily inflects the history of maternal feeling through popular genetics. Meg's generous discounting of her own maternal contribution to the
child is driven by a sense that the maternal claim to the child must reside
in one woman and cannot be shared. For Meg, however, as for the oocyte
recipients discussed in the next chapter, this singular claim is difficult to
stabilize. In what follows I consider the analysis of this difficult maternal
negotiation as a structure of feeling particular to the oocyte economy.
The properties of motherhood that are choreographed in the assisted reproductive process involve a degree of what we might term "ontological
risk," a risk to the felt unity of the maternal claim and to the desire for one's
own child (Thompson 2005).

Four. Global Oocytes

....

Medical Tourism and the

Transaction of Fertility

Assisted reproductive treatments create oocyte deficits, and once a woman finds that her own oocytes are insufficient or unviable, she may entertain the possibility of donation from another woman. Women undertaking IVF generally hope that they will provide both their own genetic material, through their oocytes, and gestational care for the resulting child. Hence the transition from IVF with ones' own oocytes to donor-assisted conception is rarely smooth. Rather, it is fraught with various degrees of grief and ambivalence, ethical compromise, rationalization, bodily risk, and logistical obstacles. The women I interviewed in Australia and Britain who turned to donation were extremely reluctant to abandon the idea that they would have a genetic relation to their children. This particular idea of motherhood, the sense that the gametes mediate the most authentic relationship to the child, is expressive of the way in which the contemporary biosciences shape the lived experience of kinship and family (Franklin 2013). Assisted reproductive technology scales up and separates the elements of female reproduction into modular, ex vivo units—stimulation, oocyte harvest, IVF, embryo transfer, and gestation—and so introduces novel forms of maternal capacity and identification. These may be genetic mother, gestational mother, or, most recently, mitochondrial mother, a status I explore in chapter 7. Each of these has an affective weighting and significance, shaped by public understandings of genetic and reproductive science and histories of ART. So oocytes may be associated with generational continuity and family resemblance, while gestation may be associated with nurture and care, although these associations are fluid, varying from woman to woman and within any given woman's self-understanding.

Each possibility for maternal identification is also shaped by regulation. Different systems of family law might, for example, define the mother as variously the woman who gives birth (Australia, the UK), the woman who provides the eggs, or the woman (the intending parent) who contracts third parties to provide each of these steps (e.g., California).[1] In some jurisdictions, mandatory donor registries enforce a certain recognition of maternal genetic contribution without an attribution of motherhood per se. Several Australian states, and the entire United Kingdom, have mandatory donor registries.[2] For some women, this obligatory form of identification is an intolerable fracturing of their maternal claim over their hoped-for child and partly informs their decision to travel overseas for donors.

In this chapter, I draw on interviews with women from both Australia and the UK who have traveled overseas to obtain oocytes. Once they had decided to seek third-party fertility, they were confronted with the absolute improbability of an altruistic donor, in the Australian cases, and the long waiting lists for "egg-share" donation in the UK. Egg sharing is a policy that offers fee subsidies to women in ART treatment who donate a proportion of their oocytes to another woman. It is framed as a way to avoid involving nonpatient women in oocyte donation, as a form of risk minimization (Blyth 2002). The British women I interviewed had contemplated egg sharing but had been deterred by long waiting lists and poor-quality oocytes. In each case, the women turned from their highly regulated national systems to overseas jurisdictions that permitted forms of transactional procurement; to Greece, Cyprus, and Spain in the case of British interviewees, and to Thailand, California, and South Africa in the Australian cases. In each of these locations, the women interviewed could rely on their comparative wealth to purchase oocytes from younger, poorer women, a political economy of which most were painfully aware. In some cases, they struggled to trust clinics and medical personnel where

English was not necessarily spoken well, and to hope that clinical standards were adequate to protect their health and ensure reliable ART procedures. In each case, they traveled thousands of miles and spent thousands of dollars or pounds, often on difficult schedules, and in secrecy from family and friends. Most of the women I interviewed did have a child in the end, and two women had twins, but not all were successful. Like many other women who undergo fruitless IVF, they then struggled to reconcile themselves with a sense of absence, of a life much anticipated but unable to be lived, the life of the never-to-be child (Tonkin 2012).

So, the procurement of third-party fertility was a painful and difficult process for most of the women I interviewed, which would describe the experiences of many women, both providers and recipients, in multiple parts of the world. At the same time, transnational oocyte markets are now a well-established dynamic in the corporate fertility sector and in the global bioeconomy more generally (Cooper and Waldby 2014). Oocyte markets have developed in several regions, for example, between South Korea (vendors) and Japan (purchasers) prior to 2008, when the Hwang scandal provoked a tightening of regulation in Korea (Leem and Park 2008).[3] In Latin America, Ecuador has developed an oocyte market featuring "light-skinned" vendors, servicing neighboring countries (Roberts 2010); and in Southeast Asia, Vietnamese women sell oocytes and gestational surrogacy to intending parents in Thailand (Whittaker and Speier 2010); while white Australian women will travel to South Africa to secure fair-skinned Afrikaans donors. In the Middle East, Sunni Muslim majority nations like Saudi Arabia prohibit oocyte donation, and couples travel to Shia-dominated Iran for donor-assisted treatment (Inhorn 2011). Within Europe, women from the northwestern member states (the UK, Scandinavia, France, Netherlands, Germany) travel to the south and east (Spain, Greece, Cyprus, Czech Republic, Russia, Poland) to purchase oocytes (Shenfield et al. 2010). In Israel in the early 2000s, fertility clinics procured oocyte donations from young Romanian women, so that their clients could avoid reliance on Palestinian women and instead source the fair-skinned "European" karyotypes that they felt better matched their own diasporic European heritage (Nahman 2013). As some of these examples suggest, oocyte procurement and patterns of circulation are frequently embedded in broader geopolitical relations. I return to Elizabeth Roberts's (2010) accounts of Ecuadorian donation and Michel Nahman's (2013) account of Israeli assisted reproduction toward the end of this chapter, as a way to tease out some of the issues of regional affiliation or disaffiliation that emerge from this study's interviews.

These regional markets give women a transactional means of obtaining oocytes. This monetized economy is partially an effect of the scarcity value oocytes acquire for women who have been through IVF, their qualities of rarity, their preciousness, and their position as the choke point in the difficult trajectory leading to the desired child. The oocyte economy is not a function of scarcity alone, however, for the demand for all types of human tissues far outstrips supply, generally speaking. Nevertheless, most national jurisdictions in industrial democracies have human tissue acts that prohibit buying and selling blood and organs, and their transfer is managed through carefully regulated gifting (Healy 2006; Waldby and Mitchell 2006). Broadly speaking, regulatory philosophies are more variable for tissues considered nonessential to the life of the donor; hair is traded across the globe with few regulatory barriers, for example (Berry 2008). Reproductive tissues are a particularly complex category in this regard. No national jurisdiction permits the trading of embryos. Indeed, since the advent of human stem cell research in the late 1990s, embryos have attracted a whole regulatory armature designed to acknowledge their proto-human status and protect them from various forms of commercialization, so that, for example, embryonic tissues cannot give rise to intellectual property in the EU (Gottweis, Salter, and Waldby 2009; Webster 2011). Oocytes are the human tissues with perhaps the highest degree of regulatory variation from jurisdiction to jurisdiction. Although in Australia, oocytes are regulated as therapeutic tissues, with strict controls around reimbursement and the criminalization of transaction, in many other jurisdictions, oocyte transactions are tolerated and coded as compensation for a gift, rather than as a fee, payment, or wage (Cooper and Waldby 2014).

This regulatory patchwork generates pent-up demand in some jurisdictions, and the possibility for supply in others. National regulators have few ways to prevent fertility patients traveling from home to a clinic elsewhere, receiving treatment, and returning home to await the result. In some cases, jurisdictions with radically opposed philosophies may share a border. Germany, for example, with its very strict approach to embryo creation and prohibition on oocyte donation, shares a border with the Czech Republic, where young rural women are paid a few hundred euros to "donate" oocytes to IVF patients.[4] For German couples seeking oocytes to drive to a Czech clinic for treatment and then drive home again a few days later is a simple matter (Bergmann 2011a, 2011b). Even between more dispersed locations, the advent of mass international travel and more widespread acceptance of all forms of medical tourism (Holliday et al. 2015), mean that fertility, like health, can be readily transacted across borders. Regional transport and service hubs like Dubai, in the United Arab Emirates, capitalized on both their location and their comparatively liberal governance to create global IVF services, attracting fertility patients from throughout the Middle East during the first decade of this century, although more recently conservative regulation has reversed this globalizing trend (Inhorn 2016). In Spain, the primary European location for transnational IVF and transactional oocyte procurement, fertility clinics have sprung up near popular tourist destinations and airports, where couples can combine a Spanish holiday with fertility treatment (Dickenson and Idiakez 2008).

In what follows I explore the experiences of nine women I interviewed, five from Australia and four from Britain, who went overseas in search of oocytes. I also draw from other fieldwork studies of fertility travel to explore and open up this experience.

Fertility Experience and the Desire for a Donor

The women I interviewed were recruited through UK and Australian fertility chat sites, with a simple posting inviting anyone interested to contact the study. In the UK cases, a broker who arranged fertility travel also assisted recruitment, contacting some of her clients and passing on my details if they seemed inclined. Although recruitment was staged over several months, with repeated postings on sites, in all only nine women came forward for an interview, a response that is perhaps indicative of the slightly illicit nature of fertility travel and its associations with eluding national regulation. In the UK group, all four were between forty and fifty at the time I spoke to them. Two were between forty-one and forty-five, and two were between forty-six and fifty. Two were married, one had a partner, and one was single. One woman had twins, two had one child, and one had no children. All had completed at least secondary education, one had a diploma/advanced diploma, and another a bachelor's degree. Their occupations were full-time mother, office manager, media professional, and bank director, and they lived in London, Essex, and Birmingham.

Of the five Australian women, one was late thirties, three were between forty-one and forty-five and one was over fifty. Three were married, one was in a de facto relationship, and one was single. One woman had four children, one had three children, one had one child, and two had no children. All of them had completed at least a bachelor's degree, and four of them had completed postgraduate studies. Their occupations were lawyer, policy advisor, economist, change manager (social media), and postsecondary teacher. The five lived in either Sydney or Melbourne. All nine women identified as heterosexual.

Eight of the nine women had long, arduous histories with IVF treatment prior to the point at which they decided to try for donor eggs. In most cases, they were in their late thirties before trying to conceive, and after six months or a year of trying through intercourse, they turned to IVF. One Australian woman had several IVF pregnancies that miscarried, while another had ten full cycles without success. The British women described delays in their access to treatment through the National Health Service (NHS), and the turn to private clinics to accelerate the process. The NHS has strict cut-off points and criteria governing access to subsidized treatment, and three of the women described variously finding their hormone levels were too low or they were too old to receive NHS treatment. Two women went on to private treatment and several cycles with very low oocyte numbers, while two others went directly to seek donation.

Olivia, a London-based media professional, and the only woman who did not try some form of treatment prior to obtaining a donor, expressed her deep regret at never trying to conceive with her own eggs. She had begun to consider single motherhood at thirty-nine. Her gynecologist advised her that she had little hope of success, and that she should pursue egg donation. In the end, her donor cycles did not work either, and she felt that in some sense this was because the eggs were not really "hers."

> I wish I'd had at least one cycle with my own eggs. I wish I hadn't given up on my own eggs quite so easily. I'd always had this mad theory— which I know has absolutely no value to it [laughs]. I discussed it with my doctor and he said that's complete rubbish—but this theory that maybe my body is rejecting it because it's not me, they're not my eggs. If it were my eggs then maybe it would have worked, because my eggs

are a part of me. I kind of wish I'd had one go, even though it probably wouldn't have worked, at least I'd know I gave it a shot. I never did give it a shot with my own eggs, so I do sort of regret that, really. (Olivia, mid-forties, single, no children, media professional)

The Australian women immediately began a search for international donation. Only one Australian woman attempted to identify a local donor, and she did this at the same time as she researched her international options. This immediate recourse to international procurement reflected the fact that Australian clinics generally do not source donors for patients and instead advise them to identify their own. Unless a woman has a willing sister or friend, their only recourse is to advertise in family-oriented print media, particularly the weekly magazines, *Sydney Child, Brisbane Child, Melbourne Child,* and *Canberra Child,* that specialized in such ads. The interviewees doubted that such advertisements would be effective and did not want to waste any more time in their bid to start a family. They disliked the ads' "desperate" tone and harbored fears about the motives of any woman who would reply with an offer of donation. The only woman to take out a print advertisement, Molly, did receive some offers, but then felt that potential donors were seeking some kind of maternal standing in the recipient family:

> MOLLY: [The respondents] sounded so needy, or almost desperate.
> INTERVIEWER: To donate?
> MOLLY: Yes!
> INTERVIEWER: What was behind their neediness, do you think?
> MOLLY: My strongest thoughts would be to latch onto another woman or a family. They just sounded needy or . . . perhaps even emotionally unstable. . . . This is my family; it's no one else's family. I didn't really want any contact. (Molly, mid-fifties, single, three children, economist)

Among the UK women, one attempted to access oocytes through the national egg-share system, while the others turned their sights overseas immediately. Leila, after two IVF attempts at an NHS clinic, was told she would never conceive with her own eggs. She turned to a private clinic in the midlands that operated an egg-share program, sourcing eggs from patients whose male partners had the primary fertility problem. She describes the experience:

> So we waited probably for about four months. We paid five hundred pounds to go on the waiting list. Yeah. So, a donor was found, and she produced I think seven or eight eggs, which I was really disappointed about, because that then gave us four eggs, after which I think three— no, two fertilized, so they were put back and that didn't work. . . . I didn't become pregnant. . . . So then, they told us that we could go back onto the waiting list, by which time the . . . waiting list was about a year, and then you would have to pay another five hundred pounds just to go back on the waiting list, and then you'd have to pay seven thousand pounds, again, which is what we paid, for another donor. So I wasn't convinced. . . . I was quite upset again about the whole thing. So, that's when I started looking on the internet to see what other people were doing. (Leila, mid-forties, married, two children, office manager)

So Leila, like the other women, began to look overseas. Her disillusionment with the egg-sharing system is common in the UK. In one study of 1,230 European women seeking overseas donation, British women cited long waiting lists and the poor quality of gametes as a major reason to travel (Shenfield et al. 2010). Another study interviewed fifty-one British patients seeking cross-border fertility treatment, and found that twenty-nine were in search of good quality eggs, citing donor shortages in the UK as their primary reason for travel (Culley et al. 2011).

The Anonymous Donor

Most of the Australian and British women explicitly stated that they wished to procure *anonymous* oocytes. This necessarily involved overseas travel because in the UK and in most states in Australia, gamete donors are obliged to register their identities and make them available to donor-conceived children once they reach eighteen years of age. Mandatory registries are designed to give children access to some specified information about their donor, which may include details about hair and eye color, height and weight, marital status, occupation, education, and health history. Children may have a right to initiate direct contact, but donors have no parental or familial rights or obligations. At time of writing (2017), mandatory registries operate in Argentina, Finland, Austria, Switzerland, the UK, Croatia, Sweden, Ireland, the Netherlands, New Zealand, Norway, and in several states in Australia.[5]

The idea of an identified donor provoked considerable anxieties among the interviewees. Molly's quotation above gives some of the flavor of this anxiety. The difficulty, for her, is the prospect of a division or dilution of her exclusive maternal claim, the idea that an identified donor might wish for a recognized stake in the resulting child. Belinda, one of the British interviewees, gives dramatic expression to this concern, when she explains the reasons she and her husband also sought an anonymous, international donor:

> BELINDA: No, we didn't [seek a UK egg donor], mainly because the . . . policy in the UK, you know, you have to— effectively, the person donating the eggs can probably claim the child back.
> INTERVIEWER: So they have to be identifiable to the child once the child is eighteen. That's my understanding.
> BELINDA: No, I believed—what we believed was that they have every right to come and claim the child back. (Belinda, mid-forties, married, one child, full-time mother)

Belinda's fear is unfounded, as donors certainly do not have legal claims over such children.

While factually incorrect, however, Belinda's fear is highly expressive of a particular kind of anxiety thrown up by the decision to procure third-party fertility, the sense that their maternal claim is not intact because of their reliance on a provider external to the family proper. She fears that her gestational claim over the child, her status as the birth mother, is no defense against the imagined superior claim of the genetic mother, and that the donor hence has a right to the child in perpetuity. She is in effect struggling to secure a stable maternal position and relation, which seems to her fragile and subject to incursion.

This fear is not idiosyncratic: a recent qualitative study of British women seeking anonymous donation found that they too were concerned about their sense of security as the mother and wished to avoid possible intrusions into family relationships (Stuart-Smith, Smith, and Scott 2012). As Erinna, one of the Australian interviewees, put it, the identified donor "becomes like a third party in your child's life," a sort of specter at the family feast. Erinna goes on to explain her concerns about the long-term consequences of identified donation, its potential, in her eyes, to disrupt her relations with her children once they reach their majority.

> I can see that there's both sides of the story: that they might want to find the mother down the track, and that sort of thing, if there's genetic disease and all those sorts of issues. But I think for the feeling of it being your child, an anonymous donor is better. My personal fear is that—I can understand that maybe the kids will blame me later on, or they'll want to look for their mother, but I think a lot of it is what the norms of society are at the time. So for decades, donors' sperm was anonymous, but now it's like people are being told, "You *should* be wanting to search for your mother," and it's almost like this obsession with the biological material as being more important than the family. So it was what I felt comfortable with, to be open with them about the process, but I just think it complicates things further if it's so open. (Erinna, early forties, married, four children, policy advisor)

So the figure of the identified donor represents a double threat: they may wish to exercise maternal rights and breach the walls of the family, and they may attract the older child away, out of the family and into the ill-advised pursuit of a chimeric genetic mother. If we consider the altruistic donor experience discussed in the previous chapter, we can see that this weighting of their oocytes, as the transmission point for maternal lineage and the absolute determinants of maternal status, is precisely the significance the donors wished to avoid. They regarded this status as an element of their gift, along with the raw material capacities of the oocyte, something they would carefully abjure so that the "true" mother might feel secure. By carefully extricating themselves from any psychological claim to the child, they sought to encourage their recipient to exercise her full claim. So we can see that the structure of feeling suggested by these concerns implies an older, pre-IVF organization of maternity, in which *biological* maternal claim could not be in doubt, even when legal maternity could be transferred through adoption. There is a sense in these feelings that maternal claim is a fixed quantity, and that the introduction of other women into such an equation necessarily dilutes and subdivides it.

Hence the women who traveled overseas were driven to shore up the integrity of the family and their proper claim to be its sole maternal figure. As Jo, one of the Australian interviewees put it,

I didn't want the issue of that person . . . being involved with me raising my child when it's technically, biologically, *their* child. (Jo, early
forties, married, no children, academic)

Jo's formulation, in which oocytes establish "true" maternity, pervaded
the reasoning of many of the interviewees. This anxiety is particularly
evident in their concerns about the degree of physical and psychological resemblance between themselves, their partners, and their child. For
these women, and in the public understanding of genetics more generally, oocytes are the biological entities associated with family resemblance
and generational transmission, and the interviews betray persistent fears
about the degree to which the child would "match" the family.

These anxieties propelled the women toward extranational procurement systems, where the provider of fertility could not act as a social
agent in the family. The women wanted to ensure that, after the oocytes
were transferred, they would be quits with the donor, in a clean, transactional exchange. Jo expresses this clearly:

We haven't considered [an Australian donor], because . . . our fertility specialist [told us about] donors having to reveal their identity, and
the child having access to that person . . . and it's really hard to get a
donor. . . . And also, going through IVF, the whole thing of producing
eggs for the purpose of extracting them for IVF, it's not pleasant, and to
ask somebody to do that, you know, for altruistic reasons or, you know,
to do me a favor, it just seemed like a big ask. And also, I didn't want the
issue of that person necessarily then being involved with me raising my
child when it's technically, biologically, *their* child, and if there would
be . . . it just seemed too messy. . . . So I thought, "Well, if I'm going to
do this, it needs to be an overseas person who basically, you know, we
cut ties with." (Jo, early forties, married, no children, academic)

Brokerage and Destination

The British women focused their search for international providers on
Europe, while the Australian women extended their search over a much
wider geography. At first glance, Europe seems an unlikely region to
seek commercial oocyte provision. EU member states are signatories to
the Oviedo Convention and the EU Tissue and Cells Directive, as well

as various national statutes that prohibit the exchange of body parts for money (Council of Europe 1997). They also belong to a broader European cultural commitment to the gift relation (Waldby and Mitchell 2006). Despite these anticommercial principles, Europe supports a vigorous intranational and cross-border oocyte market, which has developed opportunistically to exploit the discrepancies and regulatory vagaries of various member states and their neighboring jurisdictions.

In particular the market is shaped by the different ways in which member states have interpreted the European Union Tissues and Cells Directive (Directive 2004/23/EC) which forbids the exchange of human tissues for money but permits compensation "which is strictly limited to making good the expenses and inconveniences related to the donation" (Article 12[1]). Oocyte markets have developed in European states where compensation has adopted de facto features of monetization. This is evident in Spain, for example, where compensation is around €1,200 (approximately US$1,400) per cycle, paid in cash without documentation. As a consequence, couples will travel to Spain from other more tightly regulated parts of the EU, and indeed from around the world, to obtain oocytes, typically provided by students and migrants from Latin America and eastern Europe, working in agriculture or domestic service (Idiakez 2010; Bergmann 2011b). Other vigorous markets in the EU area include Greece, the Czech Republic, and Poland (Pennings et al. 2014; Alichniewicz and Michałowska 2015).

Two of the British women sought treatment in Spain, and two in Greece, while one of the latter also had treatment in Cyprus. The women related an initial enthusiasm for the United States as a destination. They were particularly attracted by the reassuring professionalism of the clinics, and the much more consumer-oriented nature of donor selection. Clients are not matched with donors by the clinic as is usual in Europe, but rather can search databases of potential donors and select not only for resemblance but also qualities like higher education attainment, musicality, and athleticism (Almeling 2011). Nonetheless, none could afford the £25,000 to £30,000 costs. All began the process through internet searches, and three eventually relied on a fertility travel brokerage, a company set up to negotiate international treatment and coordinate the complex choreography of medications, tests, and travel schedules so that donor and recipient are in the same location at the right time for insemination and embryo transfer. Brokerage is an intrinsic element in the formation of global oocyte markets, liaising between different languages and clinical systems, as well as coordinating the logistical aspects of fertility travel (Roberts 2012). Leila explains the reassurance provided by a brokerage, at a time when she felt particularly vulnerable:

> Some of the clinics looked good, but . . . it's hard, isn't it, when it's not your own language, to know they're legitimate, to know whether they're going to be at the same standard. I didn't know if they were affiliated to any kind of standard like they are in the UK: organization, regulations, that kind of thing. . . . I liaised with [an English nurse who ran a brokerage.] . . . She knew all about it, knew the staff, so that gave me some confidence because, you know, I should imagine it's bad enough going abroad to get your teeth done, but to have a baby by a woman you've never met, and to have a gynecological procedure, it's something you want to make sure it's all above board and professional. (Leila, early forties, married, two children, office manager)

While the four British women all traveled to southern Europe for their treatment, in several cases their oocyte providers were in fact East European. Olivia and Belinda, who traveled to Greece and Cyprus, had two Polish and two Russian donors, while Rachel and Leila, who went to Spain, were not informed of citizenship but presumed their donors were Spanish. The presence of East European women in southern European clinics is by now a well-documented phenomenon, reflecting both broader feminized migration patterns within Europe and the attractiveness of East European phenotypes for northern European purchasers seeking fair-skinned, blue-eyed donors (Idiakez 2010; Bergmann 2012). Women from the former Soviet Union, faced with poor employment prospects at home, migrate to the wealthier states of the European Union to supply needed childcare, elder care, and housework (Lutz 2008), or to work intermittently in the informal economy. For them, oocyte vending offers an intermittent source of additional, undocumented funds and constitutes a type of reproductive labor cognate to their other work providing nurture, care, and feminized bodywork (Cooper and Waldby 2014). A large survey of oocyte donor motivation, carried out with 1,423 respondents by Pennings and colleagues across Belgium, the Czech Republic, Finland, France, Greece, Poland, Portugal, Russia, Spain, Ukraine, and the UK, found that migrant donors were much more likely to report purely financial motives compared to those who donate within their national borders.

They also found a much higher proportion of purely transactional donors in Greek clinics (39.5 percent) than the rest of Europe, while Spanish donors reported a high rate of combined altruistic and financial incentives (56.5 percent; Pennings et al. 2014).

The British women were quite aware that their donors were in all likelihood comparatively poor and in need of money in exchange for their eggs. Leila observes that the Spanish clinics she researched had plentiful supplies of young women owing to the recession, and the comparative attraction of €1,000 for someone "on hard times":

> There was a lot of donors coming forward in Spain at that time, because of the recession, and they were being given a thousand euros in order to cover their expenses and inconvenience, which, in the grand scheme of things, doesn't seem like a lot of money really, but I suppose if you're on hard times, it's not so bad. (Leila, early forties, married, two children, office manager)

Olivia, who found her donors in Greece, had a broader knowledge of the European oocyte market, because she had researched it in her capacity as a media professional. She expressed the greatest discomfort with the process and considered it exploitative. She recalls an interview she conducted about the market:

> What really made me think about the donors is, as part of this feature, I spoke to a woman who was campaigning to try to control the whole donation market. . . . She's based in the UK—she was telling me stories. She said that most of the women are impoverished Eastern European women who want to donate their eggs either here or Europe. She said in many cases the women have been overstimulated and ended up infertile themselves. . . . It's easy to not think about it. . . . You must have to be—life must be tough if you're prepared to do that. (Olivia, mid-forties, single, no children, media professional)

The Australian women could not access a regional system in the same way as the British women. Women seeking third-party fertility are generally concerned to find a good phenotypic match, and the Australian women, being of European descent but located in the Asia-Pacific region, lack a nearby population where they might find an ethnic match, hence their far-flung destinations: two went to the United States, and one each went to Thailand, Greece, and South Africa. Jo, who traveled to Thailand, was married to a Chinese man and, of the nine women, expressed the least concern about matching. I examine her experience in more detail toward the end of the chapter.

Two women traveled to Oregon and Hawaii respectively. Miranda, a social media consultant, preferred the United States because she considered the donors better protected and less exploited than in "somewhere like . . . South Africa." She explains:

> Well, for example, part of the fees that we paid covered things like psychological and legal counseling for the donor, to make sure that at least they understood the contract, and they had thought through what they're doing. We didn't want to feel like we were exploiting someone. That was quite important. And probably my perception's totally wrong, but I guess I'd be more suspicious of that happening in South Africa, with a poorer economy. (Miranda, late thirties, de facto relationship, no children but pregnant, social media consultant)

Strikingly, Molly, who sought a donor in Greece, rejected the U.S. option precisely *because* donors were paid, a feature she associated with corporate medicine and transactional commodification of the body. Instead, she had treatment in Athens, through an egg-share program, which she considered a properly altruistic method of transferring oocytes. Of the U.S. system, she states,

> I think it's vile. . . . Children aren't a commodity. . . . So as long as [the donors] were healthy, as long as, and all the health checks were ticked over, and the, I sort of, there seems to be some evidence that empathy and generosity are partly . . . genetic . . . so that's why I chose Athens. I don't like the U.S. model. I hate it that you pay people for . . . donation. (Molly, mid-fifties, single, three children, economist)

Erinna, of German descent, traveled to South Africa to find an Afrikaans donor. She felt that their Dutch ancestry would help produce a baby that did not "look obviously different from my other children." She also reflects on the difficult ethics of payment and articulates a position somewhere between that of Miranda and Molly:

> So basically, then, you pick a donor, and how it works in South Africa—they are paid, but it's around—in our currency, I think around $1,500. Fairly similar to Britain, because I know Britain's just—with the NHS,

upped their payment to 750 pounds. So it's roughly [similar]. . . . I'd prefer to see them paid a bit more. But I guess it's that balance of not being enough so you attract absolutely desperate people, but not being so low you're not being respectful of what people are giving. (Erinna, early forties, married, four children, policy advisor)

Later in the interview, she notes that A$1,500 was worth considerably more in the South African economy, given the cost of living and that it was a "poorer country." Her donor was a small-business owner, but Erinna believed that she was motivated by payment as well as altruism, and that this was a reasonable response to comparative poverty. Erinna's preference, given the risks and the demanding nature of oocyte production, would have been to pay her "at least A$5000. We could have afforded that, and it wouldn't have been a barrier." The compensation rate was set by South African regulation, however, and Erinna and her husband were not able to pay the donor as much as they would have liked.

Jo, seeking a donor in Thailand, introduced an extra level of ethical concern, the possibility that young Thai women might be effectively trafficked into egg selling.

One thing that concerned me was that we could be unknowingly entering into some kind of black market situation, where vulnerable girls would have their bodies used by people trying to control them, but you can actually meet them, as well (Jo, early forties, married, no children, academic).

Here we can see recognition of how oocyte vending might cross over into more sinister activities in the social organization of feminized labor. Thailand, with its economic dependence on international tourism, is the site for a vigorous, poorly regulated sex work industry, which indentures young, rural women in urban brothels (Davy 2014). Jo raises the possibility that oocyte vending might also be organized along the lines of indenture, a concern that has also been raised in relation to East European egg vendors (France 2006).

These responses demonstrate a degree of empathy for the oocyte donor, a sense of cosmopolitan concern and obligation, and an acknowledgment that many donors are compelled by poverty into transacting their fertility. There is a certain kind of transnational identification here, an educated feminist sensibility that informs their concerns and shapes the approach some of the interviewees took in finding a donor. At the same time, in their quest for an anonymous international donor their articulated empathy was impersonal, procedural, and addressed more to impoverished women as a category than to any woman in particular.

The Trace of the Donor
Resemblance and Matching

When women seek third-party oocytes, they are seeking several qualities. One of these is raw fertility: the capacity of the tissue to fertilize with sperm, to unfurl the embryo, and to establish the placenta and the gestational conditions of pregnancy. Another quality is resemblance. Most are interested in concealing the absence of a genetic link to their child from any but the closest of family or friends. Hence, they are almost always driven to obtain oocytes from women who resemble themselves in some key ways. The most salient quality most women seek is ethnic resemblance; the want a donor who may be of a different nationality but of a similar phenotype—hair and eye color, skin tone, height, and weight. Beyond questions of resemblance, the women were also concerned with the donor's health status, seeking freedom from communicable and chronic disease and genetic conditions. Some actively sought an "ethical match," a donor who was judged to be competent to consent, who had her own children and who did not suggest that the two women were engaged in an exploitative relationship.

Clinics match clients with potential oocyte providers in one of two different ways. In Spain and some other parts of the European Union, clinics are required by law to nominate an appropriate match, using a codified list of qualities—height, hair and eye color, weight, skin tone, and basic information regarding educational qualifications and whether the woman had children of her own (Bergmann 2011a). Under the EU Tissues and Cells Directive (Directive 2004/23/EC), egg donation must be anonymous, and clinic control over matching is understood as a way to enforce anonymity. In the United States, Thailand, and South Africa, where the Australian women traveled, clinics presented the client with a searchable database, an annotated list of women from whom they could choose.

Three of the UK interviewees initially considered U.S. clinics, in part because they were attracted by the possibility of choosing the donor directly and selecting from both clinic panels and agencies. U.S. clinics and fertility agencies invest a great deal of effort in the curation of desirable donor panels; recruiting, testing and screening them, and ordering their phenotypic and class qualities in a standardized, searchable form that can be ranked and selected by the purchasers from among a range of choices (Almeling 2011). Their profiles might include photographs, personal statements, and information on academic and athletic achievements, musicality, religious affiliation, and so forth. More desirable profiles can command higher fees. The British women reluctantly abandoned this option when faced with the concomitant expense and turned to more affordable but less satisfactory matching processes within Europe. Rachel, who initially sought donation through the British egg-sharing system, found that it relied on a queueing ethos. She says,

> I never got that option [of a matching process] in London. I felt, when we got the call saying there was an available donor, I felt a little bit like, "Well, how is that a good donor, because you haven't asked me anything about what I want from my donor." So, I found in London they treat you a little bit like, You want a donor so much that you're going to take the next one that comes along. I felt it was a bit impersonal in London. We filled out a form. It was our height, hair color, blood type. (Rachel, early forties, married, one child, bank director).

She contrasts this with a more personalized approach provided by the Spanish clinic where she eventually traveled. She was asked to send photographs to the clinic so they could search for a match from their available pool of donors. The clinic rang soon afterward with what they described as "a really good match." I asked her what she knew about the donor. "The donor was twenty-three. A housewife. She had three children. Brown eyes, the same as me. Same hair coloring as me. Slightly shorter than me. Two inches shorter." Rachel was unsure about the ethnicity of her donor. Although the clinic was located in Spain, as we have already seen, British women will often be matched with East European donors because of a shared "fair" phenotype. Her answer indicates a residual anxiety about the degree of resemblance between herself and her child.

> I assumed she wasn't Spanish, but when you look at my baby . . . a lot of people say he looks very Mediterranean. So I don't know. That is

something I will ask [the broker]. But other people say he looks very much like me and looks like my partner. So that's not as important. It was more about characteristics, really. (Rachel, early forties, married, one child, bank director)

Leila, who had nonidentical twin boys through a Spanish clinic, also expressed anxiety about their "Mediterranean" characteristics. While she was happy with the matching process generally, she wished she knew more about the donor's family history and lineage:

I [would like to know more] about maybe her parents, grandparents, nationalities. Not that it is that much of a—you know, it wouldn't be a deciding factor, it would just be of interest, and for the boys, because now they don't know what their biological grandfather looked like. Was he a dark Spaniard, or was he English? Caucasian? Australian? I don't know. So, when I look at William, one of the twins, he's quite olive-skinned, and he's got brown eyes. They've both got brown eyes. I've got green eyes, and my husband's got blue eyes, so neither of the boys has got our eye color. (Leila, mid-forties, married, two children, office manager)

Olivia, who had three rounds of egg donation in Greece and Cyprus, was the most skeptical about the claimed thoroughness of the matching process.

My donor for that first cycle—all I knew about her was that she was Polish, in her early twenties, and the sperm donor was a Greek doctor. I had very limited information about the donors. . . . You provide photographs, and they say that they match you closely. Whether they do or not, I've got no idea—I suspect they don't. So, yeah. I was told her age, her height, her build, her eye color, her occupation, her education level, and that was the only information I got, really. (Olivia, mid-forties, single, no children, media professional)

So it is evident that, where the clinic matches donor and recipient, the women harbor some doubts about the veracity and probity of the process, even while they express a more general satisfaction. The fact of overseas travel to obtain oocytes, with their capacities to transmit genealogy and phenotypic qualities, automatically raises questions about family and ethnic provenance that, I would argue, cannot be entirely settled for women already uncertain about their maternal claims. The doubts articulated by the interviewees are expressive of the irreducible difference between normative motherhood, with the complete integration of genetic, phenotypic, kinship, and gestational capacities in one person, and the motherhood they have achieved with the aid of "foreign" third-party fertility and clinical intervention. Note that, in a cognate study of Nordic women who traveled to Spain to obtain third-party fertility, a more positive caste was given to "Mediterranean" oocytes. The couples interviewed expressed their enthusiasm for Spanish "joie de vivre"; the sunny, healthy life; the beauty of young women; and the idea that their baby might inherit a Spanish temperament—warm and outgoing, in contrast to the more phlegmatic Danish style (Kroløkke 2014). At the same time, the couples were concerned to find a good matching donor, so that the "Spanish" aspect of their child's conception could presumably be selectively concealed, a quality that possibly only they perceived.

One of the Australian women, Molly, was treated in Greece, and thus had matches chosen for her. While she was not particularly pleased with what she perceived as medical paternalism, she nevertheless was happy with the degree of resemblance between herself and her children. The other four women identified clinics in locations where they could search a database of possible donors—South Africa, Thailand, Hawaii, and Oregon. In these cases, the women seemed less concerned about the issue of resemblance, probably a result of their greater consumer agency in actively selecting a donor from a range of possible donors. In the United States, where several states have vigorous oocyte-procurement business models, clients can choose not only from the clinic's in-house donor panel but also from those of dedicated agencies, so that they can scan across quite high numbers of possible donors. Kate, who sought treatment in Oregon, describes this search process:

> Well, I first researched the in-house program at the clinic I was using, which does save a little bit of money, and usually, they're prescreened, so you don't take the risk of picking someone and having them flunk the medical. But there was no one who kind of met our fairly basic criteria, so then I researched agencies, and I settled on maybe one or two agencies based on reputation, and I mean, as with everything, there's online forums, and you can get tons of information easily. . . . Then I just spent hours and hours and hours kind of going through

profiles and narrowed it probably to ten, and then I sat down with my husband, and he ranked the ten. (Kate, early forties, married, one child, lawyer)

This form of donor identification is enabled by web-based search technologies, and it allowed the women or couple to make their selection from Australia, well before traveling to the clinic. Here we can see that donor selection partakes of the more general sorting and matching capacities that engage consumers of other kinds of online "hook-up" applications, those used for casual sex or dating, for example, ways to identify and solicit desirable kinds of strangers and initiate significant, yet limited, forms of exchange (Race 2014). The women themselves were quite alive to the similarities between these two forms of activity. As Miranda puts it,

It was a really hard decision, how to make the choice [of donor]. At first, when we saw the database, you freak out a bit because it felt a bit like online dating or something like that. Just, all these people, and you just feel overwhelmed. So then we had to come back to it later and go, "What's our criteria?" and just try to narrow it down. . . . We did have our first choice of donor, who had some hobbies which are much more aligned to mine, and so we originally chose her on that basis. She'd also done donor cycles and things previously. She wasn't available, so then we switched to the donor that we ended up using. (Miranda, late thirties, de facto relationship, no children but pregnant, social media consultant)

In notable contrast to the British women, who had no opportunity to scrutinize or compare potential donors, the Australian women described their choice process much more in terms of personal qualities and family history than degrees of resemblance. Three stated they were looking for maturity, for a proven donor, and preferably a woman who had her own children. These criteria related to the women's sense of what would constitute an ethical donation, someone sufficiently mature to make an informed decision, and someone fully aware of the somewhat onerous nature of the procedures involved. Miranda gives a good overview of the relationship between these ethical criteria:

We wanted a Caucasian donor . . . someone of medium height. I wanted someone who had had a child. . . . I'd just feel incredibly guilty in years to come if she wasn't able to have children. . . . I also wanted someone who'd done a donor cycle before. Again, they know what they're in for, so you don't feel like you're being deceptive to someone. . . . There were a few, like, twenty-year-olds . . . who we just felt were a little bit too young to make a decision like this, so we chose someone who was . . . twenty-six, so we were looking at that kind of mid- to late twenties range (Miranda, late thirties, de facto relationship, no children but pregnant, social media consultant).

Here we can see a variation on the idea that oocyte donation redistributes maternity. Miranda does not want her maternal ambitions achieved at another woman's expense. To seek an ethical donation is to respect the donor's safety and her right to her own family, as well as to protect her from coercive consent. An ethical donation will not dispossess the donor of her capacity to have children and should not proceed until she has realized her own maternal desires. That this respectful characterization of the *anonymous* donor, with its ethos of cosmopolitan feminism and procedural fairness, sits alongside the threatening figure of the *identified* donor in the interviewees' accounts is striking. This somewhat impersonal characterization of the ideal donor is also striking for the apparent lack of concern about matching. That may be because the matching process was implicit and intuitive, however, facilitated by access to photographs of their potential donors. Kate, who strongly stressed her search for an ethical donor, conceded that perhaps her resemblance-matching process was somewhat "unconscious."

INTERVIEWER: I assume you were looking for a physical match as well, to some extent? Or not?

KATE: Not initially—I should say "not intentionally," although it did turn out to be closer than I thought I was looking for, in a sense. The only physical things that we intentionally searched for was at least within an inch of my height. Shorter and taller was OK. But the eye color, hair color, things like that—religion—those were not factors for us.

INTERVIEWER: That's interesting, because they're exactly the things most people say, particularly eye coloration. It's a big selection point.

KATE: Yeah. It's hard to—I don't know if it's conscious or unconscious, because when I went to the clinic they said we did have a resemblance, and that could have been one of the reasons I was drawn to her, but I wasn't aware of doing that. (Kate, early forties, married, one child, lawyer).

Matching for the Asian Century

One Australian woman, Jo, gave a singular account of her search for an egg donor. She had made an active decision to eschew resemblance altogether. At the beginning of the process, she shared the more usual concerns regarding concealment of the donation and presentation of any resulting child as genetically "hers," and investigated clinics in Greece and the United States. She and her partner eventually decided to pursue third-party fertility in Thailand, however, with a Thai egg provider. While Jo was of European descent, her husband was Straits Chinese, and they had strong family and social links in the region. Their initial plan was to conceive a "Eurasian" child, using the husband's sperm and a fair European egg donor, but they settled eventually on trying for a "fully Asian child," an attempt in process at the time of the interview. Jo explains this decision as an extension of the general sense that Australia is *part of* Asia, evident in the large proportion of the population who are of Southeast or north Asian descent; in the general tolerance apparent in her own marriage and kinship networks; and in her wide experience of Southeast Asian travel:

> [So I went from,] "I've got to find a donor who looks like me, so nobody will ever ask!" to, "Hey, it's going to be really cool to have a fully Asian kid!" [Laughs.] . . . Why not be proud of that, and why not tell people that, and make it really obvious? I think, yeah, certainly in Australia there is much more openness in regards to the whole interracial relationships now—it's all over the place. . . . And it's just so funny that the way that we've progressed—and thank goodness we have— that when I'm in Asia, or when I'm with Asian people, there's no sense of them and me. I don't feel—I actually don't feel a cultural divide at all. . . . We tend to go to Asia when we go on holidays. . . . We

love Thailand, and we love Vietnam, and we love Singapore, and there are other places we'd like to explore, so as I said, there isn't an issue of feeling different, which is kind of nice. (Jo, early forties, married, no children, academic)

Here we can see how more general discourses about citizenship and regional belonging are in play in the domain of third-party fertility. We have already seen a version of this in the British women's preferences for EU clinics, and in Charlotte Kroløkke's study of Danish couples seeking out oocytes from southern European donors (Kroløkke 2014). These data describe the transaction of fertility between relatively similar populations, however, in a phenotypic sense, where ethnic similarity is actively pursued across the regional footprint of the European Union. Jo describes a more expansive view of regional affinity, where phenotypic differences are embraced in the interests of a sense of shared destiny, a sense widely articulated and fostered in Australian policy documents like the *Australia in the Asian Century: White Paper* (Australia in the Asian Century Task Force 2012) and in cultural acknowledgment of the importance of good links between Australia and Asia. This embrace of a visibly different lineage is particularly striking given the Australian history of fears about miscegenation and the vigorous pursuit, during the late nineteenth and most of the twentieth centuries, of a "White Australia" policy, directed primarily against anxieties about engulfment by the "yellow" races of Asia (Anderson 2005).

Here we see Jo planning her family in a fashion closer to the pursuit of mestizo hybridity described by Elizabeth Roberts in her ethnography of Ecuadorian IVF (Roberts 2012). Roberts notes the common preference for "blond" oocyte or sperm donors among dark-skinned fertility patients. They actively hope for fair-skinned, and thus beautiful, children as a result of third-party fertility assistance, rather than for children who look like themselves. This pursuit of whiteness over the pursuit of family resemblance can be explained, she argues, by the history of *blancamiento*, the whitening of the nation, as a form of national cohesion and progress, in which nineteenth- and twentieth-century elites argued for and facilitated race mixing between men of European descent and women of Indian descent. Mestizo peoples were considered the future of the nation, valued for their hybrid vigor and suitability for the Latin American continent. Roberts explains,

This racial and racist history is essential for understanding IVF in Ecuador. IVF allows its participants to be actively involved in the national whitening project through mixture. Many IVF practitioners spoke about their work as directly contributing to that project through the selection of egg and sperm donors who would *mejorar la raza* (better the race). This explicit race optimism differed from the underlying racial presumptions at work in the United States, where IVF practitioners work to maintain racial sameness. (Roberts 2012, 19–20)

While Jo is not actively participating in a positive eugenic project to improve the racial vigor of Australia, she certainly articulates her quest as an antiracist project, and with an implied affinity with emerging practices of queer family formation though visibly nonmatched adoption or surrogacy (Murphy 2013). In this, as in many respects, gay and lesbian intending parents have pioneered novel forms of family formation using ART as a way to mediate the needs of same-sex couples for access to sperm, oocytes, or gestation (Mamo 2007). A nonmatched child is here understood as simply another element in a family that embraces the signs of its nontraditional, nonheterosexual status. Jo aligns herself with this ethos, at least in its indifference to race and in its celebration of difference.

She is also explicitly caught up in a national discourse, albeit a contested one, in which the future of Australia depends on its embrace of Asia, in an economic and a cultural sense. This idea of national destiny is necessarily translated into more personal terms as the links and exchanges between the populations of Australia and East Asia become ever more dense, and as friendship and kinship networks form across this divide, as is evident in Jo's Straits Chinese–Italian family. To conceive a child whose lineage leads back into the Thai and Malay Peninsulas is simply to strengthen these networks and proclaim one's optimism for the Asian future. At the same time, her approach articulates a certain kind of assumed, postcolonial privilege, in which Thai in vivo service labor is constituted as a resource for household formation elsewhere (Cooper and Waldby 2014).

Here we can see clearly how the structure of feeling around oocyte procurement and fertility practices beautifully distills complex, longue durée social dynamics into individual desire and imagination. The rainbow family ideal that compels Jo and her partner brings with it an entire national and regional history, as well as reiterating some elements of colonial power, without explicitly invoking these large forces.

A useful counterpoint here is Michel Nahman's work on Israeli fertility practices, where we can see quite starkly how the geopolitics of the Israeli-Palestinian situation is negotiated in the clinic (Nahman 2013). Carrying out fieldwork in 2002, a year after 9/11 and amid the Al Aqsa Intifada and intensified concerns about national security and integrity, Nahman finds extensive unwillingness to procure donated oocytes from "Semitic" Palestinian women, and a strong preference, among Ashkenazi Jewish couples, for fair-skinned, small-nosed European donors.[6] The clinic where she interviewed Israeli fertility patients procured eggs from Romanian donors so that patients could conceive children with desired traits of European beauty and affirm Israel's European cultural inheritance, while enforcing the border between Israeli and Palestinian populations by refusing "Arab" eggs from an "enemy state." So here again we can see, in a much more explicit form than is evident in Jo's account, that oocyte economies play out matters of nation, race, and citizenship. Nahman puts this succinctly: "In rejecting Arab eggs, borders and national selves are made and unmade" (Nahman 2013, 127).

Divided Maternity
The Dilemma of the Informed Child

Six of the nine women interviewed conceived and bore at least one child using procured oocytes. In Jo's case, treatment was still in progress; Miranda was newly pregnant; and for Olivia, treatment did not result in a pregnancy. Consequently, most of the women had to come to some decision about what to tell their children about their parentage once they were old enough to understand. Recall that each of these women had sought overseas treatment in part to secure *anonymous* oocytes, to circumvent the mandatory registration process in their respective locations, and so to preempt the possibility that the child could seek out a particular identified donor. So the question of disclosure to the child was particularly sensitive.

There were two tendencies among the women. I would describe one tendency as the donor-conception model. This follows closely the normative position advocated by counseling professions and regulatory bodies, that being informed is in the best interests of the child in both a psychological and a medical sense. Kate provides a good account of this position, following the professional advice to give quite young children age-appropriate information rather than wait until they are more mature.

> I have books designed for little, little kids that I started reading to him—he doesn't pay attention! [Laughs.] It's one of the things that kind of resonated when we researched "tell/don't tell" was "Tell your child when they're young enough that they don't remember ever actually being sat down to be told." . . . It shouldn't be like, "When I was sixteen my parents sat me down to tell me." . . . This book is six pages long. Two giraffes who want to have a baby, and someone needs to give them a gift to have a baby! (Kate, early forties, married, one child, lawyer)

Along the same lines, Miranda states that the child has a right to know and that, when the time came, she would seek advice about the best way to proceed:

> Yeah. I'd try and get some advice there, but I think there's also a body, at least in Victoria, that looks at adopted and donor-conceived children, and I guess donor sperm has been around, and very prominent, for a long time, so I'm sure there's people out there that have got stories who can say, "Here's how we shared; here's what we feel works." (Miranda, late thirties, de facto relationship, no children but pregnant, social media consultant).

Miranda makes an analogy between sperm donation and oocyte donation, and she correctly notes that much of the body of professional advice, regulation, and knowledge derives from the much older and more widespread practice of sperm donation. The promotion of openness and the encouragement of identification in gamete donation is also a response to the shift toward identification in adoption, and a perceived history of psychological harm and medical risk to children if they are not fully informed that they have biological parents as well as social ones (Chisholm 2012).

The women who are most clearly in favor of full disclosure to the child express this implicit analogy in their own account of the *biology* of donor conception. This is most clearly articulated by Leila, who plans to tell her children she is "not their biological mummy." She explains,

> It's not like adoption, where you might feel rejected, so I'm thinking that if I just make it a natural thing that they've always known, then

it won't be as big a deal when they're older. I'm not sure at what stage I'll start saying, "I'm not your biological mummy," but I certainly will try and introduce it somehow as soon as possible. I want it to just be normal for them, rather than—and hopefully they'll be quite well adjusted and will be able to deal with it. . . . I worry about when they're at school, they might be in biology and learning about eye colors and that kind of thing, and having to discuss it with their friends that their mummy is not really their biological mummy. That's my fear. I hope they never throw it back at me. (Leila, mid-forties, married, two children, office manager)

To describe her relationship with her children, Leila draws on the language of sperm donation, where a clear distinction is made between the social father and the biological father. This distinction is clear because fathers only *ever* make genetic contributions to the biology of conception and pregnancy, and if they do not provide the sperm, their biological role is necessarily nullified. This situation does *not* describe maternal biology, however, where the woman's body provides the placental and gestational conditions for embryogenesis and pregnancy, undertakes the labor of birth and lactation, and provides the genetic components transmitted by the oocytes.

The women who were less inclined to inform their children also placed far more emphasis on the gestational aspects of maternity. Belinda expresses a somewhat conflicted claim to being the proper mother, based on her gestational role. She is unsure if she will tell her son. She asks, rhetorically,

What would it benefit the child to not be able to track down their [genetic] mother, and they don't know anybody else other than you as their mother? It's a tough one. It's a tough one. Because you've got your pictures from your first scan to that age, to whatever age they are. They don't know any different. . . . I don't know what the right answer to that is. If there is a right answer. (Belinda, mid-forties, married, one child, full-time mother)

She establishes her claim to be the primary mother through the photographic evidence of her gestational contribution, the first scan, which leads seamlessly to the first baby photos, and hence a maternal continuity between her role as gestational mother and social mother. Molly makes a much more direct and less qualified equation between her decision not to inform her child and her gestational role:

I . . . personally do not think it's essential [to tell the child]; it's not an adoption. It's a potential. And what you, your body does with it, your blood, your nutrients feed the baby; it's your baby. [My former partner] knew that right from the beginning. He had a lot of common sense for an ordinary man. And he said, "Never let anyone say it's not your child." (Molly, mid-fifties, single, three children, economist)

Conclusion

The experience of oocyte donation is intensely intercorporeal and intersubjective, even when it is anonymous. The unknown donor is personified for the women interviewed as the necessary element to supplement their own partial maternal capacities, a figure who, for some at least, threatens and dilutes the security of their maternal claim and divides their maternal identification. The women understand the relationship between donor contribution and their own gestational contribution as arrayed across a spectrum—at one extreme, Leila thinks she is not the biological mother, while at the other, Molly regards the oocytes as simply potential, which she nurtures and actuates. The women also grappled with the trace of the donor in their children, wondering if their dark eyes and olive skin might betray their donor-conceived status to others. Jo was a singular exception to this, embracing her hoped-for "fully Asian" child as a mark of pride in a progressive Australian-Asian identity with cosmopolitan values.

This intense experience of the donor as a necessary yet unsettling intrusion into the body and the family is cognate with other intercorporeal experiences evident in organ and tissue donation, where the generally anonymous donor is richly imagined and variously accommodated into the immunology of the self. For recipients of a life-saving kidney or liver, donated posthumously by a stranger, the sense of indebtedness to the donor can be quite overwhelming. The recipient may feel profound, inexpressible gratitude toward the donor, whose loss of life saves their own. They may feel that the donor's identity overtakes their own, as their immune system struggles to accommodate the foreign tissue (Waldby 2002). Donated human tissues always bear the trace of the donor, in both a histological and an individual register, and they can acquire a kind of spectral presence in which the donor's identity insists and persists in complex ways (Waldby 2000), a quality that Warwick Anderson argues is irreducible to their clinical value (Anderson 2015). While the experience narrated by the women I interviewed was not of the same magnitude as patients whose very lives were owed to others, it nevertheless conveys the women's sense that their fertile lives, and the lives of their children, would never be entirely extricated from the life of the anonymous donor. They necessarily must grapple with the implications of the donor's lineage because it has partially become their children's.

In summary then, we can see how this experience plays out historical and social dynamics that shape the contemporary organization of maternity. Biological ideas, social hierarchies, and norms around kinship, family, femininity, and maternity are lived and felt as apparently private experience. The women expressed a living negotiation with such norms and ideas in terms of their often vexed feelings about the donor. Hence, we can see that much of their anxiety about resemblance arises from the cultural value placed on a biologically integrated, fully autonomous maternity, in which the woman provides all the genetic, gestational, and care elements through her own person and that of her partner. To bear a child who is visibly at odds with this norm is to risk a loss of maternal claim and to make visible shameful debts to others. It is also to dilute and compromise the integrity of generational time, opening one's family history to the incursions of unknown others and risking their children's sense of completion and belonging. The women demonstrated various ways to interpret the relationship between the different elements and to understand the consequences of their dependence on another woman to furnish some of them. Their sense of distress was evidently sharpened by the recent regulatory and ethical shift toward identified donors, a form of donation they explicitly avoided but one that at least some of the women felt might be in their child's best interests after all.

So what we can see here is a dynamic social field around maternity, where the figure of the singular complete mother is rapidly disaggregating into several partial maternal actors, with shifting legal, biological, and social status in relation to the child and the family proper. It is, to use Williams's term, an "emergent formation," . . . a social experience which is still in process, often indeed not yet recognized as social but taken to be private, idiosyncratic, and even isolating, but which in [social] analysis has its emergent, connecting, and dominant characteristics, indeed its specific hierarchies" (Williams 1977, 132). Seeking overseas donation is one response to this volatile disaggregation, a way to reduce the potential reach of such actors, as they can be procured outside the registry systems, regulatory jurisdictions, and more customary forms of propinquity available to known donors within national space.

The historical and geopolitical specificity of this maternal norm is evident when we compare the much more capacious, less exclusive approach to donor-assisted conception among women in Ecuador, where, as Roberts puts it, all reproduction is understood to be "assisted"—by God, by family and friends, by doctors and technologies, rather than an autonomous act of the connubial couple. Here the donor is welcomed as a potential source of additional assistance, a way to make a more beautiful, fair-skinned, well-cultivated child, so that the trace of the donor is treated as a desirable quality, visible to all (Roberts 2012). Among the women I interviewed, only Jo's experience and cosmopolitan ambitions for her rainbow family suggest a similar openness to the trace of the donor, albeit an anonymous one. Her account points to a possible new variation on the theme of generational identity, a public embrace rather than a private concealment of the ways in which different genetic lineages can enrich each other. Michel Nahman's account of embattled oocyte procurement under conditions of Intifada points in the other direction, to the ways oppositional relations between Israelis and Palestinians make the transaction of "Arab" eggs impossible, as Israeli fertility patients feel obliged to guard the European affiliations of the Israeli state (Nahman 2013).

An important aspect of oocyte donation that I have not yet touched on relates to the need for synchronized cycles. The donor and recipient women have their menstrual cycles and ovulation schedules linked together by their respective clinics, in order that the recipient's body is ready to accept the embryo created by the donor eggs and partner's or donor's sperm. This clinical system effectively turns the two women's bodies into a temporarily single reproductive organism linked across space, a procedure that necessarily intensifies the intercorporeal experience of both women. One woman provides another woman with a complete stimulated cycle of oocytes, transacted fresh and in real time. These temporal and scalar features are currently being reshaped with the introduction of vitrification techniques, and a move toward corporate banking models for oocyte transaction. In the next chapter, I examine this change, and the effects of cold-chain oocytes on the experience and distribution of fertility.

Five. Cold-Chain Oocytes

....

Vitrification and the Formation
of Corporate Egg Banks

The experiences of the women who travel overseas for oocytes, described in the previous chapter, are extensively shaped by the preference for real-time and real-space transactions. Women seeking third-party fertility must travel because the donor, the intending parents, and the clinic staff all need to be in the same place at the same time. Oocytes, as a tissue, are extremely time critical, so to optimize their fertility, they are generally used fresh and transferred as quickly as possible from donor to laboratory for fertilization and embryo cultivation. The donor and recipient cycles must themselves be coordinated to maximize the chances of pregnancy. These constraints stand in sharp contrast with the circulation of semen. While some fertility patients travel to access intrauterine insemination (Andersen et al. 2009), others can avail themselves of a global export market in *frozen* semen. The most famous facility is Cryos International, the "Viking" sperm bank that sources semen from Scandinavian men and ships it around the world, to be thawed and administered at a clinic convenient for the purchaser (Kroløkke 2009). The ability to freeze and thaw fertile sperm means procurement and consumption can take place at different times, in different places, without the need for travel or for complex biological coordination between the respective parties. As a consequence, the sperm-banking model can take advantage of considerable economies of scale and a more industrial approach to human gametes than the batch-by-batch, face-to-face approach needed to manage oocytes. A new business model is emerging around oocyte donation, however, built on recent improvements in cryopreservation. Oocytes can now be banked with a certain degree of security, a development that is reshaping both local and transnational forms of oocyte provision and procurement.

As with frozen semen, frozen oocytes allow economies of scale and time management to be introduced into clinical practice. Clinics in the United States, Britain, Spain, and other locations with the right mix of regulatory liberality and donor incentives are developing egg banks as part of their service model. These are primarily in-house facilities, designed to simplify the complex art of cycle coordination and to move away from batch-by-batch transaction to more flexible, predictable, and readily packaged forms of oocyte procurement. In some cases, the new oocyte banks are following the global semen model, developing shipping systems to move frozen oocytes around both national and international space. Each approach involves a certain rationalization and depersonalization of oocyte transaction, potentially affecting the quite intense sense of the donor's identity described by recipients in the previous chapter, and foregrounding corporate dynamics in the reproductive bioeconomy. The capacity to cryopreserve women's fertility is having decisive effects on the overall shape of the oocyte economy, creating new forms of exchange, distribution, and value.

This chapter is based on twenty-four interviews with clinical, laboratory, and business staff in Brisbane and Sydney, Australia, and in Phoenix and San Francisco in the United States. It includes interviews with the directors of two egg banks: one in-house facility and one that exports oocytes around the world. These interviews were focused on professional expertise and accounts of clinical logistics, rather than on the interviewees' personal experiences. Hence, I identify each interviewee by their professional designation rather than a pseudonym. I conducted all interviews, and with two exceptions, they were conducted face to face at the relevant clinic. The exceptions were conducted by phone. I also conducted interviews at a London egg bank and will consider those data in the following chapter, which is focused on private autologous egg freezing.

Cryo-fertility
Vitrification

Cryobiology, the science of tissue freezing and thawing, has been part of the infrastructure of the biological sciences since the mid-twentieth century. Cryobiology constitutes a specialized application of cooling and freezing technologies, a set of innovations that were set in train by nineteenth-century imperial ambitions for far-flung procurement of foodstuffs, but that gathered pace with electrification and the industrialization of agriculture (Woods 2017). The repertoire of cryobiology techniques emerged in particular from the demands for wartime transportation of blood supplies for troops, from commercial food-preservation technology, and from the field of animal husbandry. Agricultural scientist Christopher Polge and colleagues, tinkering with the ratios and transportability of bull semen, discovered that the addition of glycol allowed the tissue to be frozen and thawed without loss of viability (Polge et al. 1949). This technique opened animal reproduction out to an entire infrastructure of cold storage, transportation, and various forms of "synchronization" that enabled disparate cattle herds to be inseminated by a single bull, as well as the ability to preserve genetic stock over time (Wilmot 2007b). Hence, tissue freezing emerged as a technique from a more general twentieth-century concern with the scientific management of biology and living materials, and the rationalization of both human and animal reproduction (Wilmot 2007a; Radin 2013; Radin and Kowal 2017).

Cryobiology has since become a central technique of the contemporary life sciences, as more and more kinds of tissue and cellular material can be frozen and thawed without loss of vitality. This ability to stop and start biology, to arrest and suspend cellular activity and reanimate it at some future date, involves a rearticulation of the terms of life, its given temporal pathways. As Hannah Landecker observes, biotechnology does not simply change what it means to be human; it changes what it means to be biological. In that sense cryobiology, "the ability to freeze, halt, or suspend life, and reanimate [it is] an infrastructural element of contemporary biotechnology. In short, to be biological, alive, cellular, also means (at present) . . . to be suspendable, interruptible, storable, freezable in parts" (Landecker 2005, n.p.). Landecker's point is that the ability to freeze and defrost tissues presents issues not merely of utility but of a fundamental reordering of life's trajectories. It demands that we think differently about the relations between biology and time, as well as enabling uncanny reversals and dis-synchronies. In fertility preservation, cryobiology allows gametes to outlive their donor, so that, for example, children can be posthumously conceived with a dead man's semen, with attendant social and legal anxieties about the ethics of such a practice (Kroløkke and Adrian 2013).

Until very recently, however, the secure freezing and thawing of human oocytes has remained beyond the abilities of cryobiology. Mammalian oocytes of all kinds are particularly difficult tissue to freeze because of their high cytoplasm volume and the tendency of the chromosomes lined up by the meiotic spindle to be disrupted by ice crystal formation. Human oocytes have proved more difficult to freeze and thaw successfully than those of most other mammals (Mullen 2007). Various oocyte cryopreservation techniques have been used since the early 1980s, initially developed as a way to preserve fertility for oncology patients, whose treatment often compromises their ability to have children (Kondapalli, Hong, and Garcia 2010). These initial attempts were based on techniques to minimize ice crystal formation using programmable freezers, which chilled tissues slowly (Tucker et al. 2012). The first full-term pregnancy and birth using a frozen oocyte was reported in 1986 (Chen 1986), but the success rates for ART fertilization, pregnancy, and live births using slow-freeze oocytes remained significantly lower than those for fresh cycles. Concerns were also raised regarding the safety of oocytes, which may have sustained subtle forms of spindle damage (Oktay et al. 2006).

More recently, clinics and cryobiologists have turned to the technique of vitrification, with better results. To vitrify is to transform a substance into "glass," to render it stable and inert through very rapid cooling to about −100°C, at which point molecular activity ceases. Vitrification is a technique developed first in animal reproductive biology during the 1980s (Rall and Fahy 1985) to bypass the process of ice formation that takes place during slow freezing. Ice crystal formation damages tissues because the structure of the crystal overrides the structure of the cell, and when the tissue is thawed, the cell matrix is damaged. Flash freezing, combined with appropriate cryoprotectant, generally preserves the tissue structure by lowering the freezing point and reducing the time taken to move from fresh to frozen state (Chian, Wang, and Li 2014).

Vitrification has been introduced to the field over the last ten years or so, using various protocols. A cryobiologist I interviewed at the San Francisco clinic observed that much of the early incentive to improve freezing techniques emerged from strict regulations around embryo transfer, particularly in countries like Germany and Italy, which prevented the freezing of surplus embryos.

The [IVF] regulations that came in in different countries were very different. For example, in Italy they brought in regulations that you could only inseminate the number of eggs that you planned to transfer back to the woman, so for example, if you did an egg retrieval on a woman, and you retrieved five eggs, and you inseminated all five, you had then to put all five of those back inside the woman. Even if they hadn't fertilized, you had to put them back inside her! That egg had been exposed to sperm, so that had to be transferred back to the woman. . . . So the Italians now were doubly incentivized to come up with procedures for freezing eggs, otherwise they had eggs they were just going to be throwing in the trash. . . . And there were other countries in Europe that had sort of similar restrictions. Germany had laws, France had laws, Switzerland had laws. . . . So, in the 1990s, as we went through the nineties, the number of publications on egg freezing started to go up. And in the beginning of that process, everybody was using slow freezing, and they were trying to adapt the slow-freezing process to make it work with eggs, and some people had some limited success, but nobody ever really came up with anything that caught fire, that took off and everybody started doing. But then, in the 2000s, as experience with egg freezing mounted and people were realizing, you know, "This slow freezing doesn't seem like it's going to pan out as a technology for egg freezing," people started looking at vitrification.

As various clinics experimented with vitrification protocols, some systematic studies reported significantly more success with this approach than with slow freezing oocytes (Smith et al. 2010). More importantly, a few clinical trials have compared vitrified oocytes with fresh cycles and found only slight, or no, differences in terms of fertilization and pregnancy rates (Cobo et al. 2010). After reviewing these data, both the European Society for Human Reproduction and Embryology (ESHRE) and the American Society for Reproductive Medicine (ASRM) declared that oocyte vitrification was now sufficiently advanced to no longer be regarded as experimental (ESHRE Task Force on Ethics and Law et al. 2012; American Society for Reproductive Medicine 2013). The ASRM guidelines note that the clinical trial data may not be generalizable, because of the differences between clinics in terms of specific expertise with vitrification, and the considerable variation in protocols within the technique. They also note that these success rates all relied on oocytes from young women, and that the effects of vitrification on oocytes of women over thirty-five were not fully studied. Nevertheless, the society considered the available data sufficiently persuasive to declare vitrification no longer experimental.

The implications of these declarations are considerable, signaling to the fertility sector that vitrification can now be applied to various aspects of practice with greater legitimacy. It seems likely that vitrification approaches will supplant those of equilibrium freezing in the already well-established areas of oocyte cryopreservation; for women undergoing cancer treatment, in treatment situations where oocytes are produced but not fertilized, when couples in treatment have ethical concerns about the banking of nonimplanted embryos, and where legislation forbids the creation of supernumerary embryos. The declaration is also reverberating through the nascent nonmedical, or "social," oocyte banking sector, and through clinical procedures and business models that heretofore were organized around the real-time, real-space intractabilities of oocyte transactions. These declarations effectively legitimize the various potential uses of egg-freezing services and generally boost the process of market formation.

While the clinics discussed in this chapter have offered nonmedical egg freezing since around 2008–2009, the staff I interviewed considered the declaration something of a tipping point, insofar as they reassured potential clients that they were not undergoing an experimental procedure, with its connotations of risk and uncertainty. The declarations energized discussions around the formation of egg banks, with concomitant transformations in the clinical services and business models underpinning their practice. The formalization of egg banks at each site introduced forms of corporate mediation between oocyte donors and recipients, depersonalizing the relationship to some extent and making certain kinds of risk (clinical, legal, fiduciary) more predictable and manageable. It changed how donors could be recruited, and enhanced the desirability of nonmedical egg freezing as an option for women wishing to preserve fertility into the future. The business case for a move from fresh to frozen cycles is compelling, such that almost 25 percent of U.S.

donor cycles during 2013–2014 involved cryopreservation (Kushnir and Gleicher 2016).

In the next section, I focus on how egg freezing enables the corporatization of egg donation and the development of a transnational cold chain, which may, in time, replace the fertility travel system described in chapter 4.

Giving to the Bank
Vitrification and the Corporatization of Donation

The egg-freezing programs I describe in this chapter were embedded in long-standing fertility clinics. I discuss the Arizona clinic, which specialized in both transnational and international export, in the second half of this chapter. In this section I focus on the formation of an in-house egg bank in a San Francisco clinic. The demand for egg-banking facilities at this clinic is driven to a considerable extent by its location in one of the world's most prosperous global cities. San Francisco is the corporate headquarters for U.S. trade relations with the Asia Pacific (Hartman and Carnochan 2002) and the residence of choice for the highly skilled and highly paid denizens of the West Coast information economy. One of the foremost innovation hubs in the United States, the San Francisco area attracts a well-educated professional class of managers, scientists, engineers, and venture capitalists (Storper and Scott 2009), and professional women may find that career demands, the absence of statutory maternity leave, and the extremely high costs of housing make family formation difficult. Hence, clinical fertility services find a ready market among well-educated, well-remunerated women seeking technical solutions to manage their desire for family, as well as women with medical infertility or infertile partners.

The clinic established its egg bank in 2013, and at the time of interview, it had been in operation for a little over a year. This clinic did not have long prior experience with programmable freezing and onco-fertility banking. The clinic director stated that, while they offered a banking service to adult women undergoing chemotherapy, this was a small part of their operation, and his preference was to refer such clients to university hospital-based research programs with strong links to oncology medicine and counseling. The clinic involved itself in egg freezing only after secure vitrification systems were readily available, around 2007, and it could avail itself of a skilled cryobiologist to oversee the process. Vitrification was first used for embryos, and then extended to eggs. Initially the service was slow to take off, but it now provides about three hundred freeze cycles a year, including both the donor program and private egg banking, with a steady increase each year. Growth in demand is driven by their advertising campaigns but also by the media interest in egg freezing, and by celebrity endorsements from the likes of the Kardashians.[1]

Vitrification affords the clinic an interlinking set of technical and business efficiencies. It enables a major reorganization of the temporal and social relations of third-party fertility through the process of banking. As I discuss in earlier chapters, the precise sequencing and organizing of reproductive elements is absolutely central to fertility treatment. Charis Thompson describes "synchronization" as a particular art in the fertility clinic, the expert coordination of heterogeneous temporal orders:

> In the field of ARTS, where there is a lot of ontological choreography, there are also a large number of relevant kinds of time. Devices for calibrating and coordinating different kinds of time are ubiquitous. For example, there are menstrual cycles and treatment cycles, which are cyclical and repetitive. There is the regimented, linear, and repetitive bureaucratic time of the working day into which appointments must be fitted. There is biological age—the so-called biological clock—which is linear, unidirectional, and non-repetitive. There is the time of first-person selfhood, which runs backward to cohere the psycho- and physico-biographic precursors to the crisis of infertility, makes the space of the present, and runs forward to narrate the life course. And there are the different temporal histories that different groups of patients bring to the meaning of treatment. (Thompson 2005, 10)

Temporal logistics, the practical, material organization of biological and bureaucratic time scales, are deeply implicated with affective and generational time, the time of the life course, selfhood, and family.

The ability to freeze and thaw reproductive tissues dramatically increases clinical traction over synchronization and the husbandry of reproductive potential. The cryobiologist at the San Francisco clinic noted that, in the early days of IVF, prior to secure embryo freezing, clinics were unable to manage the number of embryos created in an IVF cycle. Some clinics undertook multiple embryo transfers, with the attendant risks to maternal health and the viability of the pregnancy. At the clinic where he worked in London, during the 1980s,

> the excess embryos were either discarded or given to research, . . . even though we were transferring on day two, [the director] was still very pro-active in reducing the number of embryos that were being transferred. . . . Multiple births were always a problem, and if we ever wanted to transfer more than two embryos to anybody, or if a patient insisted on more than two, [the director] had to be consulted personally. . . . I'm still a big proponent of single embryo transfer today, and . . . we are probably the clinic in the U.S. that does the most single embryo transfers. . . . One of the reasons we've been able to [do] single embryo transfer so much is that we can freeze embryos so successfully now, so the technology has evolved to the point where 98, 99 percent of embryos that get frozen will survive.

Cryopreservation, in these terms, enables a more rational and ethical deployment of excess embryos, ensuring that they are not wasted or unwisely transferred. In a similar fashion, the creation of the egg bank simplifies the donor process and improves resource allocation, because it preempts the need to synchronize donor and recipient cycles and facilitates better batch management. It also lends itself to a more flexible pricing structure tied to tightly specified and predictable outcomes. I examine each of these effects below.

Asynchronies

Fresh oocyte donation involves finely calibrated synchronization, so that the egg provider's body is productive in the right ways at the right time, and the recipient's body is primed to accept the transfer. Once the intending mother selects a donor, their menstrual cycles are coordinated, first by "down regulating" their ovaries, arresting normal ovarian rhythms, and then a common pharmacologically ordered menstrual cycle is set in progress. The donor is stimulated to produce multiple egg follicles, and then a trigger injection sets off a sequence that enables egg retrieval. After fertilization, the recipient presents for embryo transfer three to five days later, and then hopes for a pregnancy.

So fresh oocyte transfers involve a one-to-one donation model; the intending parents select a particular donor from the panel provided by the clinic, and the donor effectively goes through the stimulated cycle on behalf of the recipient. The director of the San Francisco egg bank describes fresh cycles thus:

> You're matched up. You're going to go through the cycle at the same time as the donor, and it's a one-to-one match. . . . As the intending parent, you are going to be receiving all the eggs donated from that recipient, and those will all be inseminated with the identified partner's sperm, or sperm donor, and then those will be that intended parent's embryos. So the idea, the benefit to someone of doing a fresh cycle is that you will have all the eggs as yours for insemination, and resulting embryos. The average number of eggs that you'll find with a donor is going to be eighteen to twenty-four. . . . [O]n average our patients usually have . . . a single embryo . . . transfer, and typically will have four blastocysts frozen, so that is what the expectation is with a fresh, synchronous cycle.

Fresh donor cycles are highly personified transactions, even when they are anonymous. The pharmacological process links the biology of the donor and recipient in lockstep, effectively rendering their reproductive systems as two elements in a single, if temporary, unit. We saw some of the consequences of this intense personification in the previous chapter, where oocyte recipients were persistently troubled by their intercorporeal relationship with the donor and never felt quite free of the debt they owed to her.

The egg bank is simultaneously a legal, commercial, and technical facility that reorders this process, rendering it more corporate and more compatible with managerial imperatives and a service delivery ethos. The clinical and business personnel at the egg bank were keen to stress the complexity of developing a business model that complied with California penal and tax codes while also generating a sustainable revenue stream. The bank director explains,

> You know, building an egg bank takes a lot of capital investment. It takes a lot of—there are lots of regulations, especially in California, that have to deal with the fact that you cannot sell eggs in California, and so it took quite a while to be able to get to the point where our

legal team . . . and our financial people were comfortable with the way that we were structuring the egg bank, because there has to be different financial accounting for an egg bank than for straightforward IVF cycle, at least in California, if you are complying with the California Penal Code. So, it took a lot of investigation and a lot of investment, really, in terms of making sure that, number one, we were in compliance both with the penal code and tax codes, and then that we had a sound business model that would make it, so that we could take donors through and then be able to provide a service that would be more affordable. So, that took a number of years to develop.

The bank offers a less expensive fertility service than the personalized matching model. First, the bank becomes the contracting entity. Donors contract to supply the bank with a cycle of oocytes, while intending parents contract with the bank, not for eggs, but for a service. One of the clinic partners, an endocrinologist, explains the promise enshrined in the contract with patients:

> What we do is promise them the service for cost, and then we promise them that they'll achieve at least two transferable embryos for the fee that they pay. And if they don't, then we do it over again. So that's worked out well, and the attorneys tell us that it's legal and can be done. We're not selling eggs; we're providing a service that uses the eggs, and some financial protection for patients that they're going to get at least two transferable embryos.

The bank employs the language of service to avoid possible infringement of the California Penal Code, which explicitly bans the transfer of "any human organ, for purposes of transplantation, for valuable consideration," but excludes from "human organ" plasma, sperm, and any other renewable or regenerative tissue not otherwise specified (Cal. Penal Code §367f [2011]). Whether this ban extends to oocytes is not clear, and the sector has adopted "compensation for services," rather than "payment for tissues," as a framing device to avoid direct contravention of the law (Terman 2008). While clients would pay US$35,000 to US$45,000 for a fresh, fully matched cycle with disposal over all fertilized eggs produced, the egg bank service guarantees two viable embryos for US$21,000 (prices at time of interview, 2014). This enables the clinic to offer a more affordable "family-building service" to couples wanting only one, or one additional, child. Couples who want two or three children who are genetic siblings are advised to contract a personal donor and create embryos from all the viable eggs, while the bank offers a better route for others.

Banked eggs, however, placed the risks of donor recruitment and embryo creation squarely on the clinic, because to accumulate inventory, bank staff had to identify desirable donors' profiles themselves and proceed with stimulation. In the case of fresh cycles, the more personal matching process ensured that the commissioning couple would selected the donor prior to the recipient's entry into treatment. As the director of the bank explained to me, this redistribution of risk meant that it was unwise, from a risk-management point of view, to build too much inventory. She asks, rhetorically,

> How much capital do you want to invest, and how much capital do you want to have sitting around as frozen eggs? . . . We're very selective in terms of our donors. . . . So, it's a combination of, How many donors do we want to run through in a month? And then, Are there that many donors that really meet our criteria? I mean, you want to have enough inventory for people to have a choice. You want the inventory to be matched, because if you invest in a donor, and her profile is not appealing, or something else is not appealing, and she doesn't match, you're not going to get a return on your investment in terms of your cost as a clinic, or as a bank, to have her go through IVF. . . . When you do a fresh cycle, there's no investment on the clinic's part. The fees that are paid to the donors are passed through, as it has to be, legally, in California. . . . But here, we are putting all this up front. . . . We're paying to run the donor through. We're taking on the risk. We're hoping that she's an appealing donor, so that there will be matches made by intended parents there.

So egg banks assume the matching risks, and the San Francisco clinic rigorously screens a high volume of potential donors to accept less than 2 percent of initial applicants. Those who proceed to provision for the bank must have excellent genetic and somatic health, family health history, high levels of fertility, a desirable phenotype (which might include women of East Asian, African American, and Hispanic origin as well as white European descent), and the capacity to score highly on complex psychological tests that screen for qualities like emotional stability and mental health issues like depression and anxiety.[2]

Each of these screening steps adds costs to the clinic, and each donor represents more of an investment risk. Yet, the bank also extracts more value from each donor cycle, because it exploits the *divisibility* of frozen oocytes. Fresh eggs, because they are time critical, cannot be readily apportioned among different recipients. The labor-intensive nature of synchronous cycles, and the extremely fine temporal adjustments required to bring donor and recipient into alignment, means that a cycle of fresh eggs cannot be parceled up into smaller units. Only one recipient can be synchronized with one donor, and fresh eggs need to be quickly fertilized if any viable embryos are to result. Hence, intending parents necessarily contract for the entire cycle of eggs, and may consequently end up with several frozen embryos that they are unable to transfer. Frozen oocytes, on the other hand, are not time critical. The entire raison d'etre for cryopreservation is the suspension of biological processes, its removal from the temporal constraints that condition fresh tissues (Radin and Kowal 2017). Frozen oocytes can be disaggregated from their batch and diverted one by one along different temporal and social pathways. One clinician, an endocrinologist, explained the advantage of frozen eggs over fresh as related to "efficiency," a term that implies the improvement of input-output ratios and the elimination of waste.

> It's mostly an efficiency issue, where a donor will generally produce an excess number of eggs, more than anybody could possibly use, and to be able to split those among multiple recipients reduces the cost, is really what it comes down to. It is certainly possible to match recipients to work with a fresh donor, but as you can imagine . . . to try to split a fresh donor and get everybody's cycles matched up, and evenly split the [cycle,] it's a challenge. So, in our view, we couldn't really do that cost effectively. . . . So to be able to put those eggs in the freezer and just have them there, and then pull out a batch of . . . six or eight eggs at a time for an individual patient, basically doing an asynchronous cycle. You know, the recipient gets ready at a separate time than the donor, which has proven to be much more efficient, and it's lowered the cost. We have an outstanding lab. We're getting very, very good pregnancy rates with that process.

So while the egg bank transfers recruitment risks onto the clinic, it also rationalizes the biological vagaries and intractabilities of the assisted fertility process and facilitates a more efficient monetization of egg cycles and embryo creation. Less clinical time is needed to coordinate cycles, and fewer eggs can be used to make more viable embryos and distribute them to more families at a lower entry-level cost. The manager of the egg bank estimates that for each donor cycle, which might produce twelve to twenty mature eggs, three sets of intending parents can receive viable embryos. So we can see the decisive effects vitrification has on the logistics of the oocyte economy. As it becomes more reliable and a more mainstream approach to oocyte procurement, management, and distribution, oocytes lose a degree of their scarcity value, and the intractable material quality of the tissue is modified into more calculable terms.

Depersonalization

At the same time, this divisibility removes the highly personalized, one-to-one nature of egg donation. We saw in chapter 3 that, for the altruistic Australian egg donors, the known status of the recipients was crucial to their sense of purpose, their understanding that they were helping in the formation of a happy, caring family. While I did not interview any U.S.-based donors, I did ask clinical and counseling staff about their perceptions of the donor's feelings about giving to a bank rather than to a specific woman or couple. Note that the donor program for both fresh and banked eggs at this clinic is entirely anonymous, so donors and intending parents cannot opt to meet one another or exchange identifying information. The typical donor profile was a woman in her early to mid-twenties, with a bachelor's degree, often involved in postgraduate studies and often in a clinical profession, particularly nursing. The egg bank patient coordinator noted that nurses were attracted to the notion of service and interested in scientific innovation, and this predisposed them to egg donation to some extent. She indicated that some potential donors had a strong preference for matched donation, while others were more agnostic:

> Some donors like the idea of having a match between a one to one. We've noticed that from the donors that have experienced fresh cycles. . . . So there is a transition period where the donors that were selected for the donor egg bank had [already] done cycles with us, so it is a different experience to say, you know, "You are typically selected.

You're selected by somebody." Donors like the idea that someone liked me, someone liked my profile. "I've been selected!" They often want to know—there's a question in their application, a question for intending parents, and they say, "Why did you select my profile?" and we do ask for the fresh program, for the intended parents, we ask them to write a letter to the donor, because the donor doesn't get to learn anything about the intending parents. The intending parents get to learn a lot about the donor, because obviously they get to see the profile. So the letter's really nice for the donors to feel like they're doing this for a person, they're doing this for people that have chosen "me." . . . It personalizes the experience. We noticed with the donors who had done . . . the fresh synchronous cycles, when we started talking to them about doing the donor egg bank . . . the difference in the program is that you will not receive the letters. The timing is . . . very difficult, because frozen eggs can be frozen indefinitely, and even though the donors are thinking about this right now, those eggs could be selected three years, five years down the track, when their life could have changed. So . . . for some people, that's very important. They'd prefer to stay in fresh [donation], and they'd prefer to do a one-to-one donation, where they have more of an idea of that connection.

So we can see here an affective investment broadly similar to that of the altruistic Australian donors, a desire, despite anonymization and the transactional nature of the process, to establish a connection with the recipient woman or couple. At time of interview, the clinic had around fifty donors listed for fresh matched cycles, and about thirty donors with a cycle of vitrified eggs in the bank, a distribution that reflects not only the preferences of the donors but the more rigorous risk-managed approach to the accumulation of vitrified inventory. It seems likely that, despite the reduced medication regime and less stringent compliance demands of bank donation, many donors will continue to prefer a matched process, with its sense of direct, personalized, and embodied contribution to the creation of another's family.

In summary, at the San Francisco clinic and other similar in-house banks, vitrification was used primarily to manage *time*. Banked eggs are a far more tractable resource than fresh eggs, more readily accumulated, rationalized, divided, and allocated, precisely because they are not time critical. Unlike fresh eggs, their value does not have to be spent immediately and all at once, but rather can be preserved and realized egg by egg. Vitri-fication allowed the clinic to dispense with the rigors of the synchronized cycle. The biological time of donor and recipient women no longer had to mesh precisely, nor did they need to be coterminous. As the patient coordinator noted above, a vitrified donation may not be used for several years, but rather remain as "latent life" (Radin 2013) awaiting the interest of an intending parent sometime in the future. Given the fragile, time-critical qualities and powers particular to oocytes, this new technical capacity represents a decisive shift in how women's fertility can be ordered. I take up this theme of time and oocyte banking in the next chapter, "Private Oocytes," which examines the more experiential and affective dimensions of this new technology as a way to preserve personal fertility.

Cold-Chain Fertility

Cryobiology offers important ways to manage and reorient *space* as well as time. In this section, I consider the development of *export* oocyte banks, facilities that transport eggs through both national and international space.

The history of cryobiology is the history of preservation *and* transportation. Much of the early impetus for the science of cryobiology came from the demands for plasma transportation during World War Two. Blood products to treat battlefield casualties had to be kept stable through not only refrigeration but also mobile forms of packaging, insulation, and shipping that could maintain a stable low temperature across long distances, and through variations of ambient temperature, humidity, and power supply (Radin 2012, 2013). The idea of the cold chain combines the practices of storage—preservation in time—with those of distribution through space. Secure cold chains are central to significant sectors of the food and chemical industries, where freshness and viability of product is determined by precise kinds of mobile refrigeration. In the biomedical sector, secure cold chains, with carefully calibrated procedures for point-to-point transfer, are particularly important for vaccine manufacture and distribution, where small variations in humidity and temperature can compromise potency, and hence the immunity of the vaccinated person. Cold-chain security is also central to most forms of tissue banking. In the case of biologicals, like tissues and vaccines, the material is not only temperature stabilized but also tracked and validated, monitored and handled according to protocols and good manufacturing practice (GMP) regulation, and in compliance with the requirements of bodies like the U.S. Food and Drug Administration (FDA), Health Canada, the European Medicines Agency (EMA), and the World Health Organization (WHO) (Castiaux 2011).

The reproductive medicine field involves specialized forms of cold-chain management because of the widespread use of low-temperature forms of cryopreservation to transport embryos, sperm, and now oocytes. The complexities of the cryogenic cold chain are such that logistics companies like Cryoport specialize in the transport of semen, embryos, and other reproductive tissues around the world, using dry vapor dewars, liquid nitrogen, insulation transport, tracking technology, chain of custody documentation, and an entire suite of logistics to ensure the preservation of fertility across space.[3] The demand for these services is increasing as reproductive markets become increasingly globalized, and more and more gametes and embryos are transported from place to place. So, for example, the Cryos bank, mentioned earlier, specializes in the curation of desirable genetics from a relatively remote geographical region, Scandinavia, with its associations to clean living and tall, fair, educated masculinity, and exports them to less well-endowed regions of the world. The centrality of cold-chain logistics is inscribed in the bank's title (*cryos*, "ice"). From Denmark, the company exports to seventy other countries, using proprietary cryoprotectant and packaging, as well as standardized protocols and quality assurance processes that can be licensed to other banks. Kroløkke notes the play on Viking virility throughout the bank's marketing, including the equation between legendary seagoing prowess and Cryos's efficient shipping protocols (Kroløkke 2009). The growth of international surrogacy is also driving the expansion of the cryogenic cold chain, as intending parents send their gametes or embryos to India or Thailand for gestation and birth, and even commission gametes from a third location to be shipped to the clinic managing the gestation (Lee 2009).

The transportation of frozen semen is a well-established practice, and many corporate sperm banks have several years of operational experience to underpin their quality assurance. The protocols for the semen cold chain are relatively standardized, and particular clinics have developed proprietary systems that stabilize their accumulated experience and provide a degree of certainty about the efficacy of their product as it moves through space. While oocyte vitrification is becoming a more and more common service in clinics, a very small number of clinics currently attempt to ship oocytes through space. This is not only a technical matter but also a matter of negotiating different regulatory regimes, as vitrified oocytes travel from one zone of governance to another. While transnational reproductive travel is a method that largely eludes regulators, this is not the case with transnational oocytes. In what follows, I describe the small but growing U.S. export sector and look in more detail at the part of this industry that exports beyond North America.

Export Oocytes

In 2013 seven oocyte banks in the United States shipped eggs elsewhere, as distinct from clinics that included in-house vitrification services (Quaas et al. 2013).[4] Four were exclusively focused on the national fertility market, exporting only within the United States. Two banks exported vitrified oocytes to Canada amid some controversy, as it is unclear how the U.S. system, which allows payment for oocyte donation, interacts with the prohibition on payment that characterizes Canadian regulation (Downie and Baylis 2013). Since 2013, the sector has expanded, although in the absence of central registries, the number of export clinics is unclear. At the time of my U.S. fieldwork (2014), only one bank exported beyond North America, and this is my focus here. Its business model is particularly interesting because of its negotiation of the regulatory barriers that stand between the frank contract market for oocytes in the United States and the regulated gift regimes characterizing the bank's two major destinations: Australia and the United Kingdom.

The bank is based in Arizona, in the Southwest United States, and has developed from an earlier oocyte brokerage company. The brokerage sector works alongside the clinical sector in the United States, particularly on the West Coast, and allows clinics to outsource their donor recruitment to specialists who focus on matching donors with recipients and on managing the contractual aspects of the process (Almeling 2011). The bank initially opened its doors in 2004 using slow freezing and switched to vitrification in 2009. The bank's approach to donor remuneration is comparatively flat, as it does not engage in packaging donor characteristics (education, beauty, etc.) for higher fees. At time of interview (2014), egg providers were paid between US$3,500 and US$5,000 in addition to reimbursement of costs, which falls well within the ASRM guidelines (Ethics Committee of the American Society for Reproductive Medicine 2007), but is rather lower than the estimated national average of around US$10,000 per cycle (Levine 2010). As I discuss below, this flat rate approach to remuneration has proved an advantage in the export market.

The bank head office is not a physical bank but the coordination point for a set of retrieval centers and the cold-chain process that underpins its export model. Retrieval clinics are dotted around the West Coast and the Southwest. The bank headquarters focuses on donor identification and recruitment, while the retrieval centers carry out the stimulation, retrieval, and vitrification of the eggs for transport. The laboratory director of one retrieval clinic on the West Coast noted that this dispersed system of clinics expands the bank's access to different phenotypes, in her case, to young East Asian women.

> [The bank has] a donor egg registry, so they recruit from . . . mostly Arizona, and Indianapolis. But if they get someone who inquires, or if they have a recipient—for example, if they find that someone in Australia specifically wants an Asian donor, Arizona is not a good place to get an Asian donor; nor is Indianapolis. But here is. So, we do primarily Asian young women who have been designated as an egg donor for a particular person someplace else, like Australia. So, we would create the—we would do the stimulation on the donor, get the eggs, freeze them, and then we ship them off to the bank, to their headquarters, and they store them and disperse them to whomever.

As the laboratory director's words suggest, the bank does not accumulate inventory as an in-house bank does. Rather the donor panel is listed on the bank website, and once a couple selects a donor, she will begin hormone treatment and retrieval from one of the bank's clinics, who ship them on. The bank's CEO explained the reasoning behind this model:

> It was a decision I made a while ago that I didn't want to bank a lot of donor eggs because technology changes, and I didn't want to have old technology for people, because that would really present a financial and ethical dilemma. . . . So basically, people can go to our roster, and in the U.S. there are about 450 donors on our roster of donors, pick

four or five, and call us up, and we help them through the matching process. . . . And people are allowed to meet the donors they like, and talk to the donor with us on the phone. So, once the donor is selected, then we take first the egg retrieval.

So in the first instance, the bank provides an asynchronous cycle of oocytes that can be shipped to intending parents within eight weeks of matching. The retrieval clinics are the first point in the cold chain and must ensure that their flash-freezing process preserves the integrity of the oocytes and readies them for transportation. The bank has assembled considerable expertise in reproductive cryobiology, and their scientific staff train personnel at the retrieval clinics. Recently, they have filed patent on a cold-chain technology.

Since 2013, the destinations for vitrified eggs have included a chain of fertility clinics in the UK and in Australia. At first glance these import arrangements seem highly improbable and in breach of regulation. Both statutory and administrative law in Australia and in the UK forbid the exchange of human tissues, including oocytes, for money, and the UK is also bound by EU directives to that effect.[5] The bank, however, following the usual U.S. model, pays its donors, albeit within the ASRM guidelines for reimbursement. Moreover, the UK and most states in Australia have mandatory registries for gamete donors, discussed at length in chapter 4. No similar registration requirements operate in the United States, and no commercial oocyte bank releases donor identity in the normal course of events (Quaas et al. 2013). Both the UK and some states in Australia stipulate that patients must receive formal approval from the regulator to import gametes from overseas, and all applications are scrutinized to ensure that they conform to state and national legislation, including the reimbursement of donors.[6]

So on face value, the possibility to export U.S. oocytes to Australia and the UK seems closed off by several layers of regulation, including mandatory identification and criminal sanctions around the exchange of human tissue for money. In practice, however, the UK regulator, the Human Fertilisation and Embryology Authority (HFEA), and the Australian state-based regulator, the Victorian Assisted Reproductive Treatment Authority (VARTA), which has a similar mandate to the HFEA, have moved toward a certain liberalization of these constraints, in response to pressures exerted by the vigor of the transnational fertility travel sector. This is particularly evident in the UK, where the HFEA launched a public consultation on donor compensation in early 2011. The consultation document listed the HFEA's major concerns as the shortage of domestic donors, long waiting times for treatment, and the risks to British fertility patients if they use web-based matching services or overseas services, including poor care in unlicensed clinics. In other words, the consultation was concerned about how transnational fertility market pressures affected British patients. In October 2011, a directive was added to the Human Fertilisation and Embryology Act 1990, which increased allowable compensation rates for oocyte donation from £250 to £750, as well as reducing the amount of documentation required to receive compensation. This, in effect, brought the UK donation system much closer to the Spanish one, in an attempt to neutralize Spain as the destination of choice for UK fertility travelers by expanding the number of domestic donors and the national supply of oocytes. We can see here how the terms of compensation are adjusted and expanded to manage the demand pressures created by both national waiting lists and transactional oocyte markets elsewhere (Cooper and Waldby 2014).

In Australia, there has been no similar move to introduce undocumented reimbursement or to provide incentives for donation. Yet, VARTA has publicly expressed concern about the medical and ethical risks to Australian fertility patients traveling to clinics in South Africa or Southeast Asia to purchase oocytes (Victorian Assisted Reproductive Treatment Authority 2012). One Australian clinical director, whose clinics are currently involved in importing vitrified oocytes from a U.S. bank, confirmed that VARTA had worked with her to identify ways to import gametes, as a measure to reduce Australian fertility travel and to protect the well-being of patients:

> Well, what started the whole process was a real desire to try and find some supplies of eggs, because we were really quite desperate. . . . I had been helped a little by the fact that VARTA had determined some ways and rules which they thought may assist in determin[ing] if it was feasible to bring gametes from commercial banks into Australia. What was starting to concern us a great deal was, a number of our patients were actually going overseas for treatment . . . to South Africa,

a number to Spain, some to the U.S., and then some starting to go
to Thailand. . . . We have heard horror stories of some of the consequences of care in some of these countries.

Hence, the negotiation of oocyte importation from the United States has
proceeded in a climate of regulatory uncertainty as to how to respond to
the domestic pressures created by the international fertility market, and a
certain willingness to explore options that once seemed outré.

Offshoring Regulation

The arrangement between the Australian clinic and the U.S. egg bank
involved protracted and complex negotiations between all the parties.
After making initial contact in 2011 and taking legal advice, the Australian
clinic organized a series of meetings with the Reproductive Technology
Accreditation Committee, which oversees clinical practice, licensing, and
auditing of the Australian fertility sector; the Australian and New Zealand Infertility Counselling Association; and VARTA, which would oversee
any egg importations into the state of Victoria. U.S. bank representatives
were also invited to key meetings to work out the import-export pathway.

The result of these negotiations is a dedicated program within the
U.S. bank that fully complies with Australian federal and state-based
legislation, accreditation processes, and practice guidelines. The bank
recruits and screens a pool of potential donors who are prepared to provide oocytes without the usual U.S. fee. In the case of the UK, donors
may receive the equivalent of £750 (about US$1,000) above and beyond
documented expenses, but in Australia, they may be reimbursed only for
expenses incurred, including time away from work, babysitting needs,
costs to attend the clinic, and so on. To meet specific Victorian state legislation, the U.S. bank's counselor is registered with the Australian and
New Zealand Infertility Councillors Association (ANZICA) and follows the
Australian clinic's procedures for the psychological evaluation of donors
as well as briefing donors on the regulatory requirements of an Australian donation. This includes preparing donors for identity registration
and possible contact by any children conceived once they reach eighteen
years of age. The donors have a second counseling session, on Skype,
with an Australian clinic counselor, and if they proceed to donation, they

must met Australian federal and state consent requirements. Once they have moved through these compliance points, they are made available to Australian clients as donors. The U.S. bank forwards not only the frozen oocytes but also the extensive paperwork needed to verify expense claims as well as counseling and consent procedures, and these documents become part of the Australian clinic's compliance audit.

The arrangement has been struck by, in effect, including the U.S. bank within the Australian federal and state regulatory footprint. The bank has been constituted as a regulatory outpost, a location that complies with the requirements of the various Australian regulatory bodies, despite being located in another national space. Hence, it can retrieve and export oocytes through a tightly managed transnational trajectory, which involves not only advanced cryobiology techniques but also point-to-point transport of clinical ethics, mandatory documentation, identity verification, and a precise counseling ethos. This strategy represents a particularly complex example of the development of bilateral and multilateral regulatory harmonization between clinics in different jurisdictions as a way to manage the forces of fertility tourism, an approach advocated by VARTA (Victorian Assisted Reproductive Treatment Authority 2012). The Australian Reproductive Technology Accreditation Committee (RTAC), which licenses Australian fertility clinics, has developed an international accreditation and quality-assurance scheme to facilitate such standardization, and they are in negotiation particularly with clinics in Southeast Asia. The Thomson Fertility Centre in Singapore is the first such facility to receive RTAC accreditation so far.

The striking feature of the Australia-U.S. agreement, however, is the negotiation of highly regulated, altruistic, identified donation within a U.S. system associated with transactional procurement and the absence of statutes. The U.S. bank's comparatively conservative approach to compensation, and its adherence to the lower end of ASRM guidelines, has made it a less improbable partner with UK and Australian clinics than fertility brokers in California, New York, and some other states that pursue high-fee, niche-market business models.

At time of interview, the U.S. oocyte bank had approximately 150 women who had agreed to be considered for the Australian and UK donation program, from a total of about 450. These are clearly small numbers when compared to the numbers of women and couples who travel overseas to obtain oocytes. The Australian-U.S. program can only address a very small corner of this overall demand. Its significance, however, extends well beyond its particular operation. First, it represents a form of cross-border fertility transfer that does not set out to elude national regulation. While transnational fertility travel relies on various national regulators' inability to govern clinics and patients beyond the borders of their jurisdictions, the Australia-U.S. program remains within Australian national jurisdiction despite its international scope. It increases Australian patients' access to donors without the need for travel and while remaining within a precautionary gift system. Second, it represents a new business model for gamete banking. The agreement negotiated between the Australian clinics and the U.S. bank has cleared a path with the regulators for other agencies to pursue similar bilateral or multilateral agreements, as well as laying out the steps needed to do so. The agreement has forged a specific path through a thicket of regulation and technical constraints that other agencies might follow. It seems likely that other Australian and British clinics will want to pursue similar arrangements with overseas oocyte banks, to stay competitive and to meet patient demand. The extent to which U.S. oocyte banks can recruit a significant pool of altruistic donors within a commercial contract system remains to be seen, however, and this may place significant constraints on future arrangements. This bilateral and multilateral strategy may also create implicit pressures for the harmonization of compensation regimes, as is evident in the UK de facto adoption of the liberal Spanish approach to compensation.

Conclusion
The Regulatory Cold Chain

Vitrification is an important technical development in the social management of oocytes, but it will not, in itself, shape the social relations of fertility that might develop around this innovation. Rather these will be shaped by the regulatory landscapes through which cold-chain oocytes travel, and the kinds of constraints and protections for both donors and recipients that they encode. The case I have focused on is notable because it creates a regulatory chain to supplement the technical cold chain: a trail of documentation, licensing arrangements, and compliance procedures that meet the ethical criteria set out by the importer jurisdiction. Hence, while these cold-chain oocytes "travel alone" across borders, they travel through a regulatory trajectory that has been carefully constructed between their point of embarkation and their point of arrival. If more such bilateral and multilateral arrangements are created, the kind of chain involved will depend on the regulatory ethos of the respective export and import jurisdictions and the pathways that are negotiated between them. Cold-chain oocytes present an ethical advantage in the sense that they are much more readily regulated than the movement of fertility travelers themselves, assuming that enforceable regulations exist and clinics observe them in good faith.

Vitrification is having some decisive effects in the oocyte economy and in its value hierarchies. This chapter has examined the logistical dimension and the political economy of these effects, the material leverage that egg freezing gives over earlier time and space constraints on the clinical management of women's fertility, and the ways in which this conditions the value form of the oocyte economy. Freezing is an innovation that stabilizes not only the biology of oocytes, their fertile capacity, but also their commercial status. Frozen oocytes can be accumulated as inventory and more precisely monetized, so that new pricing structures and affordability niches can be introduced into fertility clinic services. The elimination of the finely calibrated, time-critical, personalized nature of fresh cycles means that frozen inventory is far more predictable, more modular, and more anonymous, although of necessity, oocytes must convey the genetic trace of their provider. The bank's curation of its donor panel represents a more explicit human capital investment than the method of fresh cycle matching, because each donor involves more potential risk and hence demands more fine-grained selection and cultivation. For donors, too, the act of provision is more akin to a professional service than a personal relationship, a transaction with the bank rather than a (remunerated) gift to a deserving infertile couple.

In the next chapter, "Private Oocytes," I focus on some of the affective and experiential dimensions of egg freezing, the structure of feeling organized by the emerging practice of "social" oocyte banking.

Six. Private Oocytes

....

Personal Egg Banking and
Generational Time

Cryopreservation and the creation of corporatized egg banks are having a distinct effect on the oocyte economy. Vitrification introduces multiple efficiencies and logistic flexibilities into this economy, giving clinics and banks much more control over the procurement and matching process. The ability to bank oocytes means that fertility can be accumulated, organized through material inventories, retained through time, and shipped through space. It allows for time lags between procurement and provision, and the subdivision of batches among different recipients. These logistical advantages also introduce a different dynamic between donor and recipient, rendering the relationship less intensely personified. The donor gives not to another woman but to the bank, and her eggs may be preserved for months or years before they are matched with a woman seeking treatment. The donor and recipient cycles are not synchronized, and hence they are not locked into each other's biology and embodiment in the same direct fashion. For some donors at least, this less personal relationship was felt as a loss, and they elected to remain in fresh provision and synchronized cycles, despite more onerous and inflexible schedules.

In this chapter I investigate another cryopreservation option now available to women: private egg freezing. In what follows I am less concerned about the logistics and more concerned with the affective dimensions of egg banking. How does the ability to preserve personal fertility through time shape how women think and feel about their fertility generally and their oocytes more specifically? In considering this I do not comment on the extent to which women who use private egg banking are misled by the fertility sector, an objection that has attracted a large commentary literature (see, for example, Shkedi-Rafid and Hashiloni-Dolev 2011; Mohapatra 2014). Rather, I draw on interview material to consider what this new technical capacity to arrest the flow of fertile time tells us about the structure of feeling associated with the oocyte economy.

Private, or "social," egg freezing, as it is sometimes termed, describes a service in which women bank their eggs for later use in conceiving a child. It is the most recent addition to a whole suite of personal tissue-banking services, where clients preserve their own tissues for future use (Waldby 2006). A significant segment of private tissue banking is focused on reproductive tissues and the preservation of personal reproductive capacity through time. Women may variously bank their child's cord blood (Brown and Kraft 2006), their IVF embryos (Nisker et al. 2010), their menstrual blood (Fannin 2013), or their breast milk (Ryan, Team, and Alexander 2013), while men may bank semen, if, for example, they are facing a tour of duty in the military or a gonadotoxic cancer treatment (Johnson et al. 2013).

Personal reproductive tissue banking values the tissue in a particular kind of way. Clinics provide a highly individualized service to women who attribute their own oocytes with unique, nonsubstitutable qualities. In the exchange market for third-party fertility, discussed in chapter 4, allogeneic oocytes have a primarily instrumental value for the woman who obtains them. They are the means to produce the long-desired pregnancy, and the fact that these allogeneic tissues transmit the genetics of the provider is something to be tolerated, concealed, and treated as the price paid for the priceless child. This recourse to third-party provision also has emotional costs, the sense that provider genetics override the recipient's maternal contribution. Some recipients felt that they were, in some sense, maternal imposters.

The appeal of private egg banking arises from a similar cluster of feelings about the importance of nuclear genetic relatedness. Yet it presents a different solution. It inverts the transactional dynamic associated with third-party fertility, avoiding exchange and placing the highest value on the fact that banked oocytes are the transmission point for the client's own unique genetic material. Matthew Chrulew argues that cryobiology's capacity to freeze genetic codes and their potential constitutes its most significant affordance, a capacity he explores in relation to endangered species preservation (Chrulew 2017). His point is equally applicable to private tissue banking, which is organized to value personal genetics above other possible biological qualities and to retain this personal value against the depredations of time. Private cord-blood banking, for example, is organized to retain the neonate's genetic material, despite the availability of public, allogeneic (donated) cord blood banks with proven therapeutic efficacy (Brown and Kraft 2006; Waldby 2006).

Here we can see that both eggs and cord blood can be ordered *either* according to their exchange value, where self-identical genetics is less important than clinical efficacy, *or* according to their singularity value. I use the term "singularity value" in the sense developed by Lucien Karpik (Karpik 2010), to describe the value of nonfungible goods, those that have a unique incommensurable status. They are not subject to the laws of general exchange and price equivalence that govern the circulation of commodities. They are goods that, for the consumer, have no quantifiable equivalence or tradable value. They are goods—Karpik uses the examples of works of art, haute cuisine, and personalized professional services, among others—that are nonstandardizable and whose value pertains to the benefit they confer on specific consumers, rather than to their general exchangeability. For the women I interviewed about the decision to bank their eggs, their singularity inhered in their unique genetic signature, an entirely personal quality that they attributed with the highest importance. Nolwenn Bühler, in her analysis of public understanding of egg freezing and fertility extension, notes that oocytes are increasingly involved in mainstream understandings of family descent and genealogy, in part as an effect of these new techniques, whereas historically, the transmission of family genetics was associated with sperm and masculine agency (Bühler 2015). Certainly, the women involved in this study evinced a highly articulate sense of the centrality of their oocytes to the continuation of a genetic legacy, and to the ordering of their place in generational time.

In what follows, I draw on interviews I conducted with fifteen women who had banked their eggs, and with ten counseling, clinical, and business staff who worked at two fertility clinics in London. While the National Health Service (NHS) provides publicly funded fertility clinics in the UK, the two clinics here are private, and they place a premium on client choice. The NHS subsidizes egg freezing for fertility preservation in case of cancer treatment, a practice known as medical egg freezing. "Social" egg freezing designates a practice that is treated as elective within NHS guidelines. It is classified as medically unnecessary, an effect of patient or consumer choice. Hence it does not attract a subsidy, and the service is offered entirely in the private sector.

Nonmedical egg freezing is still a relatively boutique aspect of fertility treatment. In 2016 seventy-two clinics in the UK offered egg freezing, up from thirty-five clinics in 2014.[1] These high numbers, however, are not necessarily indicative of high levels of nonmedical freezing at each clinic. The HFEA, in its 2016 annual report, notes that eight clinics performed half of the total storage cycles for 2014, while most other clinics performed fewer than ten cycles each (Human Fertilisation and Embryology Authority 2016). The HFEA reports that in 2014, 816 women undertook nonmedical egg freezing, a significant increase from 2013, when there were 652 women. This reflects an annual increase of about 25 percent per year since 2010. In 2014, 129 women actually attempted to use their frozen eggs. Since 2001, fewer than sixty babies have been born to UK patients storing and thawing their own eggs (Human Fertilisation and Embryology Authority 2016).

The clinics chosen for this study were approached because they have significant egg-banking facilities and comparatively long-term experience (five years in one case, ten in the other) with slow-freezing and vitrification techniques, compared to the rest of the sector. The total clientele for nonmedical egg freezing at the two clinics numbered around two hundred at the time of interviews (2013). The clinics advertise the service on their websites and include egg freezing among the topics covered in their regular single women's seminars, which are advertised on the London underground and in other public spaces. One of the two clinics was in the process of developing a formal egg bank, analogous to its successful sperm bank, and a public advertising campaign was planned around the launch of this facility, targeting egg donation and social egg freezing. Clinical staff also noted that social egg freezing had become a popular topic in both the human interest/women's sections of the news media and in high-end women's magazines, for example, *Vogue* (Hass 2011) and *Grazia Daily UK* (Shane 2012), a phenomenon that in itself provoked many inquiries to the clinic.

In this chapter I am interested in how those who bank their oocytes make sense of and use this technical capacity as an aspect of their fertile life course and personal biography. How does the technical ability to preserve fertility through time interact with quotidian and qualitative understandings of time and with different trajectories—of career, relationships, aging—that interweave at different rates through the life course? What does it tell us about the significance of fertility, and the lived experience of the repro-genetic sciences? What does it add to our understanding of the structure of feeling that is generated around the contemporary oocyte economy?

The Fertility Cliff

Egg freezing is an expensive, elective medical procedure. As such, most of its clientele are from a particular demographic: well-educated single women in their thirties and forties with high disposable incomes. This demographic is well represented in London (Skeggs 2004), and some of the drivers that propel women into freezing their eggs relate to the sexual politics and political economy of London as one of the great global cities. Since the 1980s, London has been at the forefront of urban globalization, with city and national governance that favors flexible labor markets, along with high levels of mobility and global commercial competition, particularly in financial services, the culture industries, and the knowledge economy (Syrett and Sepulveda 2012). It is a magnet for a highly credentialed professional workforce, and like other such global cities, well-educated women are attracted to the employment opportunities and service cultures these cities offer, yet at the same time, they struggle to reconcile the demands of professional expectations with those of household formation and childcare (Zimmerman et al. 2006). London is also historically at the forefront of new forms of consumption and markets for niche services, including personalized medical services (Karpik 2010), and is a major center for biomedical research and advanced clinical expertise (Lucci and Harrison 2011). The proliferation of fertility clinics in London is testament to these dynamics, taking advantage of the British leadership in reproductive sciences (Wilmot 2007a) to translate laboratory science into advanced client services.

The women recruited for the study belonged to the professional class described above. They were aged between twenty-six and forty-five, with most (80 percent) over thirty-six. Only three women were under thirty-five. All were well educated, with either a bachelor's degree (60 percent) or a postgraduate degree (40 percent). All the women were professionals. Their occupations included a personal assistant in the financial sector, a police officer, a human resources professional, a charity association professional, three business owners or managers, a commercial lawyer, an occupational therapist, a project manager, an engineer, and three media professionals. Four of the women had a longer-term partner, two were in relatively new relationships, and the rest were single. One woman was in a same-sex relationship, while the others identified as heterosexual. One woman had a child and one was expecting, and they had in both cases conceived without use of their frozen eggs. One woman was from a south Asian background, while the rest were of western European descent.

For most of the interviewees, their initial knowledge of egg freezing came either from print media coverage or from the experience and knowledge of their peer group. When made aware by the experience of friends, either a friend had investigated egg freezing directly or had age-related difficulties with conception. Participants spoke of friends who had miscarried, who had sought sperm donation, and who had been through IVF.

INTERVIEWER: How were you aware about fertility decline in the second half of your thirties?

PHOEBE: I think actually it's not something that's generally spoken about, and I think I didn't really know a lot. It was just something I had heard. . . . I have friends who've had children in their forties and I'm kind of aware that that's the last window. One of my really good friends, actually, she'd gone through IVF at the age of forty-four, and because of her age she actually went for egg donation, and she went to Cyprus last year to do it, and she asked me to be her support person.

INTERVIEWER: Oh! Did you go to Cyprus?

PHOEBE: Yes. In summer last year, and that was really good, I think, for opening my eyes about how the procedure worked . . . [and] last year I went to a few information evenings, and I didn't know the actual statistics until they were put in front of me, and I just thought, "Oh, my god, that's so scary!" Like, every year matters, you know? (Phoebe, late thirties, engineer)

Phoebe is referring to the statistical analysis known as the "fertility cliff," the probability that women's fertility will decline precipitously in the second half of their thirties (Faddy 1992). This truncation of fertility in the late thirties was felt to be quite out of step with the women's sense that they themselves were not "old":

I thought about it [egg freezing] maybe for half a year, and I was thirty-nine then. I'm now forty, and I thought, "Well, I read that by forty your fertility's declining." . . . My grandma, she had a child in her forties. So I'm not concerned about myself—I wasn't—but I thought I'd just go and see someone. . . . When you turn forty, even though I don't feel forty, it is kind of a society [pressure]. I think it was more outside influences than an internal thing, "Oh, I'm getting old!" It was more like that thought, "Well, I'm told I'm getting old, so I better do something now! (Ava, early forties, media producer)

Stopping the Biological Clock

The participants found the idea of aging eggs incongruous with their experience of themselves as youthful, as though their eggs and the rest of their bodies were on two quite different schedules. The idea most commonly used to describe this was that of the biological clock, ominously ticking at a rate that seemed at odds with other rhythms in their lives:

I think the problem is that women are not made aware of their biological clock, and they're not routinely tested for that. But that probably doesn't apply to every woman. . . . But I certainly think that if you're thinking of delaying it, you should check, you should be encouraged to check out what your parameters biologically are. (Jennifer, early forties, company director)

The attraction of egg freezing was precisely its promise to synchronize their biological clocks with other time lines in their life course. Cryobiology enables complex forms of synchronization, bringing together carefully timed, discretely preserved elements—frozen sperm, frozen embryos—in precise combinations, that would otherwise move along intractable, incompatible trajectories (Thompson 2005). For the women I interviewed, egg freezing offered the possibility that the apparently inexorable, accelerating decline of their fertility could be brought into a better, more appropriate relationship with the biographical time of their life course, running both backward into personal history and forward into hopes and plans.

This quality led Naomi to describe egg freezing as "banking time." Speaking of her sense of pressure to find a relationship, she stated,

> I was getting anxious. I felt out of control, especially the fact that I was single and all that. . . . [With egg freezing] I just felt like I'd bought some time, I'd done all I can. You've banked some time. (Naomi, late thirties, recruitment consultant).

Naomi felt she had diverted her fertility from its otherwise intractable trajectory, storing it to be redeployed at a more opportune time. Michelle commented on the uncanniness of such an arrangement, the division of self into frozen and nonfrozen parts.

> It's a bit odd, isn't it, thinking, "I've got a part of me frozen somewhere." I found that at bit odd, and then I'm thinking, "Alright, so essentially I've got to pay rent every year [laughs] to keep it!" It's quite a bizarre process. It's not something you do every day. But mentally I was, oh, I've got a back-up now. It's quite a nice feeling, in a way, that you've got that option. (Michelle, late twenties, police officer)

This capacity to synchronize different temporal strands of their body's physiology, however, was not simply an issue of pragmatics or logistics. Rather, as Thompson suggests regarding IVF treatment generally, it had complex implications for the way they could redeem their pasts and envisage their futures (Thompson 2005).

Sexuality and Household Formation

The participants wanted access to their fertility after they had established a stable household, with a reliable, trustworthy partner. They reported the difficulties of securing a relationship, and the prohibitive expense of the London housing market, as the two aspects of life inimical to childbearing at this point in their lives. In most cases, they reported a long-term relationship during their twenties and early thirties that had come to an end, leaving them with the problem of identifying a partner interested in children and the creation of a stable family. Here the dynamics of the global city, with its mobile young professionals and rapid inflows and outflows of expertise, worked against the interviewees. The ubiquity of internet dating, and the problems specific to this technique, thematized the difficulty of reconciling the churn of quick turnover relationships in the anonymity of London with the urgency of dwindling fertility:

> I went through a point [of internet dating] where I was doing so many. . . . One internet date that went on any longer than a second date, it was a guy that I saw for three months, and. . . . it just felt relaxed. It just felt like two people connected. And so . . . yeah, but it turned out he was seeing—he was seeing three other people. So this is the thing. You don't really know who you're meeting. (Anita, early forties, small-business owner)

Several of the women stated that they had banked their eggs primarily to take the pressure off their relationships with prospective partners. The quick turnover effects of internet dating, the pressure it put on the parties to evaluate each other, the difficulty of establishing trust in the absence of context—all these aspects of online dating were rendered more acute when considered from the point of view of dwindling fertility. Several stated that they feared forming an unwise relationship if they did not do something to gain more time. Louise saw egg freezing as a way to *redeem* the time she spends as a single woman, and to use it wisely, rather than impetuously invest it in the wrong relationship:

> Being single for five or six years, I thought, . . . I'm wasting all this time. I don't want the pressure of feeling I've got to settle down, I've got to have kids, and everything's got to happen so quickly, because what I was realizing from dating is that it takes a long time to get to

know somebody. Most of the time, when you have relationships in your teens or your twenties, you're working together, or you're living together, a small group of people, so you get to know people in many varieties of situations over time, and it's easier. It's not like that in your thirties. You're internet dating. It's very much dinner dates. It's one to one. It's quite intense. You have to be a very good judge of character. So for something to happen, I was like, "Well, if I'm not going to do anything about this, I'm going to have to meet someone and get married and have a baby within two years of meeting them, and I just felt that was too much pressure. (Louise, late thirties, PA, finance sector)

It is evident that egg freezing is commonly caught up in a particular kind of heterosexual romance, one in which women hope to secure an ideal future family along relatively normative lines. In contrast, one of the interviewees, Phoebe, an engineer, identified as lesbian and was in a relationship with another woman. The London clinics involved in this study had a strong consumer focus on gay and lesbian couples, with dedicated treatment tracks that facilitated oocyte donation between partners as well as sourcing sperm donation, to give each partner a biological role in a pregnancy, for example. These innovative uses of assisted reproduction, to reorder biological constraints and create new kinds of genetic affinity are signal qualities of LGBTQ engagement with the technology (Mamo 2007). Phoebe's reasons for egg freezing were in part about preserving the ability for mutual biological (genetic and gestational) relations with the pregnancy and child, but they were also caught up in broader concerns about how to negotiate the early days of a new relationship, and a sense that it would remove a certain kind of pressure on a tenuous situation.

> INTERVIEWER: Did you discuss [egg freezing] with the new partner?
> PHOEBE: No. I went to the information evenings without telling her. I just felt like it was really early to talk about anything like that. Also, too, I just thought maybe we'll break up next month. . . . I know that things can change really quickly sometimes unless you know someone very, very well already. So yes, I did that without speaking to her about it, and I don't think I'd even told her I was thinking about it. (Phoebe, late thirties, engineer)

So for both the heterosexual and lesbian interviewees, egg freezing was a way to ensure that they were not "wasting time," that is "fertile time," while they sought a partner and pursued household stability. Egg freezing was invested with the redemptive power to render both past and future as meaningful and valuable, rather than as time lost or wasted. Here the power to synchronize meant that fertile capacity could be stopped at a viable point, while other strands of the life course were ordered into line.

The Ovarian Reserve Test
Calculating Fertility Futures

Clinic staff informed me that most women approach the service to have their fertility clinically evaluated, as a guide to deciding between several different courses of action. For most of the women I interviewed, their level of fertility was unknown and untested, and my interviews with clinical staff confirmed that this was the most usual situation for their egg-freezing clients. In the words of a clinic nurse, "Those who come for consultation [want to] . . . check to see how fertile they are, how much time they've got left, do they really need to do it, and how much is it going to cost, and how many times, that sort of thing. So they're really gathering information. They haven't quite made up their mind."

Women who seek IVF treatment generally have several years of bitter experience with nonconception or miscarriage that informs them that they or their partners have suboptimal fertility, but for women seeking egg freezing, this is not the case. Among the women I interviewed, while two described earlier failed attempts to get pregnant, the most usual life trajectory was the use of contraception during their teens and twenties to prevent conception, only to find themselves in their mid- to late thirties without a partner. Their knowledge of the statistical decline in fertility during their thirties is gleaned from popular media, but the state of their own particular fertility is entirely opaque.

Clients seeking such knowledge are tested to establish what is termed the "ovarian reserve," the number of primordial oocyte follicles detectable in the ovaries, as the best indicator of overall fertility. The two clinics involved in this study used three main methods to determine ovarian reserve: they measured serum levels of follicle-stimulating hormone (FSH) and anti-Müllerian hormone (AMH), as well as scanning the ovaries to do a visual antral follicle count. The tests, however, like all medical tests, are constrained and shaped in particular ways (Waldby 1996). While they produce metrics of various kinds, they do not constitute a transparent representation of the woman's fertility. Nevertheless, the various results are combined to give the consultant expert guidance in advising the woman about her current and future fertility. Most waited anxiously for the test results. Naomi and Meredith expressed this anxiety eloquently:

> I was very, very nervous because I knew at that point that they were going to do a test to find out if I was fertile, and I was like, "Oh, my god, this is going to be life-changing for me if I can't." In a sense, I was having to deal with that, that I'd left it too late. (Naomi, late thirties, recruitment consultant)

INTERVIEWER: OK. So, were you—did you feel kind of anxious waiting for the test results? Or were you fairly calm about it?

MEREDITH: Uh, . . . yeah, a little bit, I suppose, because, well, things like the ovarian reserve, it's quite a big determining factor of your future, isn't it. It's one of those things that you can't really change. So I have to get on with it. Yeah. It was nice, actually. It was good news when it came through. (Meredith, early thirties, occupational therapist)

Phoebe reported similar feelings of trepidation:

INTERVIEWER: Did you have the test when you presented to the clinic to tell you what your fertility level was?

PHOEBE: [Yes the] AMH test that you can get. It came back really low. I was like, "Oh, damn. I'm too old. I waited too long." I've had one egg collection so far, and they got about thirteen or fourteen eggs. (Phoebe, late thirties, engineer)

So for Meredith, the test was measuring her future possibilities, and the results confirmed that she had reason to hope. For Phoebe, the test results suggested that she was too far along the declining curve of fertile life, yet these results proved somewhat misleading. She had one cycle of treatment and retrieved an encouraging number of eggs. She plans to have further cycles.

In the clinical setting, the ovarian reserve tests are designed to give patient and clinician a metric for future fertility, and to introduce a degree of calculative rationality into what until then had been experienced as incoherent anxiety and a subjective sense of lost time. Poignantly, as this clinician observed, poor test results can themselves *exacerbate* a sense of lost time.

> People who freeze their eggs tend to think there's absolutely nothing wrong with them, and for some of them it's a real shock when the egg quality is [poor]. . . . You've made that decision. . . . You're empowered into thinking, I'm going to do this, I'm not going to worry about it. But then you have your AMH test and it makes you [start] thinking, what have I done with my life? (Patient coordinator and embryologist)

Test results are not simply decisional devices for the women seeking to preserve their fertility. While they introduce some quantified, objective information into a situation heretofore experienced as personal and opaque, the interpretation of their meaning for the woman being tested is inflected through a complex and deeply felt field of desires for the future and regret for time past. For this reason, the result did not determine the subsequent course of action. Of the fifteen women interviewed, one-third reported a "low" count, while the remaining women reported average or good. In all cases, they proceeded with egg banking. Clinic staff confirmed that women interpret the significance of the test results in idiosyncratic ways, so that a low result might be taken as a reason to proceed, while a high result might be treated as a reason to postpone. While in some clinics, the decision lies with the consultant, these clinics insist on the woman's ultimate right to decide, irrespective of the result. In the words of one staff member,

> Our clinics are patient-focused clinics. . . . If you know you've got a negligible chance of success with your own eggs, but you just want to try before you think about donor eggs . . . for lots of women, you just need to try. And you take that control—and equally, you can take that control and say, "No, the odds of my treatment working are so small, and if it does work, the risk of miscarriage or whatever are increased." (patient counselor)

So while the ovarian reserve tests constituted decisional points, the decision itself emerged from a complex sense of personal biography, and how the women understood their body's history and future possibilities.

The Future Family and Generational Time

At one level, egg freezing is a highly rational strategy for management of the life trajectory. In one light, it could be framed as a form of instrumental consumer risk calculation, another example of the entrepreneurial subject of commercial medicine (Rose and Novas 2004, Waldby 2006). Such an analysis, however, would ignore the poignant, deeply felt ethos each interviewee brought to the issue, and, more tellingly, the way egg freezing involved a refusal of more pragmatic, efficient reproductive options. The *noninstrumental* kinds of value they attributed to their banked oocytes are striking. Rather than a biomechanical means to ensure pregnancy, egg freezing was discussed as a way to *defer* attempts to conceive, to create a margin of deliberative time in which to sort through different options for the future.

> I thought the least stressful action would be to discuss various options, and thought, well, we'll freeze my eggs. It's taking the stress out of the situation, really, more than anything else, and that will give me time to sort out [what I want]—it's very stressful. You can't—my body's not going to wait, is it! (Jennifer, early forties, company director)

The participants described the process as buying time and keeping certain options in play that would otherwise have been foreclosed by dwindling fertility. So for Ava, freezing her eggs did not necessarily commit her to one course of action or another; *rather it kept several courses of action and forms of future open at once.*

> It wasn't that I was trying to have a baby. . . . It was more like for security, I guess, because we all get older. And since then the weight [is off my shoulders]—I feel much more—I don't know if the pressure has become less—finding, or even looking for someone, I'm just happy the way it is, and if things fall into place then this [using the frozen eggs] won't be an option. Or maybe it will, but at least I'll have something. (Ava, early forties, media producer)

For the women, the primary value of retaining their own eggs was their promise of genetic *continuity* (Bühler 2015), and the ways in which they positioned the woman in *generational time*. As I outline in chapter 1, the gametes are the cells that inherit and transmit the history of former reproductive relations and link past generational time with future generational time (Margulis and Sagan 1986). They communicate a particular *provenance,* an accumulated history specific to themselves that confer their auratic singularity (Benjamin [1935] 1968). The women discussed in chapter 4 who sought egg donors, were haunted by the sense that the donation invalidated this generational link with the child, that they were not the real mother but a pretender.

It was precisely this sense of provenance the women who froze their eggs wished to preserve. When I asked them if they would consider oocyte donation from a younger woman, participants were generally negative. Jennifer's comments are representative.

INTERVIEWER: Did you ever think about a donor egg?

JENNIFER: I just don't think there would be any point—I can't see the point. I mean, you might as well adopt. . . . You don't know what you're going to get, do you? [Laughs.] You don't know what you're going to get with yourself, at the best of times! So no, I wouldn't do that. I mean, I'm not having a child—I'm not having it just to have a designer child. I'm doing it because I would like a child myself; I think most women . . . would have chosen their own egg over a donor. [I think] . . . genetics play quite a strong part in personality and character. It's fascinating. Which is why I wouldn't have a donor. (Jennifer, early forties, company director)

Jennifer wants to conceive with her own oocytes because she wants to maintain the genetic relation with the future child, as well as the gestational relationship.

The logics of generational time were also evident in the ways many of the interviewees evoked their own happy childhoods and families in their thinking about egg freezing. They sought continuity, the ability to re-create and transmit this form of household intimacy. In Louise's words,

Well, I think I always assumed I was going to have a family. My parents are still together. I had a very good, happy childhood and upbringing, and I had long-term relationships all the way through, from teenage until thirty. My last relationship was five years long, and the end of that we were engaged, and I always assumed that. . . . I was going to get married and have a family. (Louise, late thirties, PA, finance sector)

The desire for continuity was also evident in the frequency with which parents, particularly mothers, offered support and attended clinics and surgery with their daughters as they went through the process. In five cases, families contributed money, paying for either part or all of the procedure. In these cases we can see that egg freezing was regarded as a way to enable family continuity, and the transition from one generation to the next, a technology so valued not only by the women but by their parents.

Participants also desired a genetic relation with their future partners, not a relation of *descent* but a horizontal genetic relation, in the sense that they wished for their *combined* genetic contribution to the conception. Most of the participants had not actively entertained the option of sperm donation to conceive a child or to create and bank embryos. Four of the women acknowledged that they were prepared to consider sperm donation if they could not find the desired partner. With sperm donation, the woman is committed to single motherhood, and any resulting child would be her genetic offspring but not related to any future partner. For the single lesbian respondent, this desire for a horizontal genetic relation was also in evidence. Phoebe planned to donate her oocytes to her partner if the relationship were to coalesce around a desire for children, so that each woman would play a directly biological reproductive role in conception and gestation, and each woman would partake of the same genetic material.

Conclusion

So, in summary, what does the new oocyte tissue economy made possible by nonmedical banking mean to the women who use this service? Women use egg freezing to reconcile otherwise incommensurable differences between the time scale of their reproductive biology, the steadily elongating nature of the life course, and the increasingly iterative structure of portfolio careers and relationship formation. These differences involve not only the instrumental calculation and management of time, its allocation among competing priorities, but also *the value and meaning of time*. While the women interviewed habitually resorted to the *motif* of the biological clock, I would argue that the analogy is inadequate to the experience it is deployed to describe, precisely because of these issues of value and meaning. Clock time ticks away in regular increments, each the same value as the last, equalizing one moment to the next and organizing time in an instrumental, homogenous forward flow. For the women interviewed, however, their sense of urgency arises from the way the loss of fertile capacity steadily accelerates, compounding loss on loss, so that the sense of *lost time* becomes more and more acute and compelling.

This cascading loss forced an acute awareness of how egg freezing could potentially redeem both past and future, by arresting fertile time, stabilizing its power to create new lifetimes. Once stabilized, they hoped to better synchronize the otherwise conflicting time scales that shaped and constrained their lives. Here the synchronic arts of the IVF clinic have been extended beyond the logistics of in vitro fertility into a more general social space. Women purchase this synchronic power not in the service of immediate conception, but as a way to create a margin for deliberation and relational negotiation, without the ever-accumulating pressure created by dwindling fertility. The women needed this margin so that they could grapple with their place in the flow of generational time, and as the best way to ensure family continuity in both genetic and social senses. Their actions were not prudential but hopeful, oriented to the creation of future possibilities for life and family.

Seven. Innovation Oocytes

....

Therapeutic Cloning and
Mitochondrial Donation

Oocytes are understood to redeem and transmit time: the time of the life course, if they can be mobilized before they lose their reproductive powers, and the flow of generational time. Their reproductive capacities are both fragile and miraculous, time critical and yet temporally expansive. Carefully deployed, they can unfurl the genetic and affective history that is each woman's provenance and propel it into the future as a new lifetime and line of descent. In this sense they repay a felt sense of indebtedness to previous generations and fulfill obligations to the future.

These capacities for generational renewal do not exhaust the temporal versatility of oocytes. I touch on this expanded sense of temporal action in chapter 1, where I describe how oocytes are now essential elements in experimental biology and at the leading edge of biomedical innovation. As Sarah Franklin argues, the now widespread applications and variations of IVF technique, its status as a platform technology, have potentiated the entire biology of human and animal reproduction: "One way to view the history of IVF is as a basic technique that has circulated through science, medicine, and agriculture as part of an increasingly complex tool kit for the control of mammalian reproduction. From this point of view, the history of IVF is that of a stem technology that has become ever more thickly imbricated in the remaking of the biological that so distinctly characterized the twentieth century—a model technique for remaking life" (Franklin 2013, 2). This platform, the general application across a wide variety of fields and innovation areas, provides the technical conditions for the potentiation of oocytes, the way in which the biological and clinical sciences gain access to their capacities to reset the initial conditions of reproduction. Hence the new oocyte techniques enable the science of animal reproductive cloning and of patient-specific stem cell lines, or therapeutic cloning. In their different ways, these techniques reverse the developmental process of the organism, returning its apparently dedicated and individuated existence to its pluripotent embryological state. They run the organism back to its single-cell origins and regain the open developmental possibilities presented by totipotency, the point at which the cell can set the entire creature in train.

This ability to reiterate ontogenesis is now finding applications in herd and domestic animal reproduction (Murray and Maga 2016), and in human biomedicine, where stem cell applications have the potential to regenerate damaged organs and tissues. The latter is a development I examine in more detail in this chapter. In an even more speculative realm, these oocyte techniques are at the center of bids to redeem and reverse evolutionary time, the loss of species in the past and present. Various research programs around the world are focused on attempts to reverse species loss by reviving endangered, recently lost, and even long-extinct creatures, using similar techniques to those used to now clone agricultural animals. Endangered species are cloned in zoological programs (Friese 2013), and attempts have been made to clone variously the thylacine, the mammoth (Shapiro 2015), the passenger pigeon (Jørgensen 2013), and doubtless many other extinct creatures.[1] These de-extinction gestures depend on the generative capacities of oocytes for their plausibility. Without mammalian oocytes to unfurl ancient or endangered genetic material, the imagined world of future wildlife and revitalized ecosystems could not be sustained. Oocytes are assumed to have the power to regenerate nature as well as human health, to reverse extinction as well as clinical degeneration, indeed to reverse and regenerate biological time, restoring animals and human patients to a former, if imagined, integrity.

In this chapter I also examine another aspect of human oocyte innovation and temporal biology, the development of techniques to transplant mitochondria. I discuss in chapter 1 the ways in which oocyte biology leads back into the deep time of mammalian evolution, and even further into the life of the earliest biota. The legacy of evolutionary time is conserved in the structure of the egg and transmitted through its organelles and cytoplasm. The most highly conserved organelles are the mitochondria, transmitted down the female line without modification. This transmission may, however, involve serious pathology: mitochondria play an important part in general cellular metabolism and function, and if they are faulty, they may transmit illness and disability from mother to child. Many clinical programs around the world diagnose and treat the symptoms of mitochondrial disease, which include strokes, seizures, gastrointestinal problems, blindness, deafness, heart and kidney problems, muscle failure, heat/cold intolerance, diabetes, immune system problems, and liver disease. At time of writing (2017), however, there was only one program, in the north of England, actively focused on prevention through mitochondrial donation.

Women with healthy mitochondrial histories are asked to donate their eggs to women with family histories of disease, and the recipients' nuclear genetic material is transferred to the healthy egg. This enables the recipient to conceive a child who is genetically her own, if the terms of genetics are limited to nuclear DNA. This process is of particular interest to the current study because it gives insights into how the different components of oocytes are understood, and how their different temporal capacities play out.

Each of these therapeutic practices relies, however, on the provision of oocytes, and as with reproductive provision, this need creates a choke point. Women have proved largely unwilling to donate oocytes for blue-sky innovation like therapeutic cloning, and this unwillingness, and the fundamental difficulties of the bench science, has limited somatic cell nuclear transfer (SCNT) research to a tiny handful of laboratories. Since 2013, some of these have succeeded in creating human SCNT embryos, but interest in the field has waned and diverted to the ethically and logistically less difficult induced pluripotent stem cells (iPSCs). Mitochondrial donation evokes a different kind of donation dynamic, as it is more directly therapeutic. At time of this writing, the Newcastle University scheme was recruiting mDNA donors, and they hoped to treat up to twenty-five mitochondrial patients per year.[2]

Pluripotent Time

Somatic Cell Nuclear Transfer and the Problem
of Oocyte Procurement

In chapter 1 I give an account of how oocyte biology underpins the process that produced Dolly the sheep, and many other mammals since. Dolly's birth in 1996 effectively rent a tear in the fabric of biological understanding, because she demonstrated that the arrow of biological time no longer traveled irrevocably forward (Franklin 2007). The SCNT process effectively uses the inherent capacities of the oocyte to reverse engineer biological development. It takes dedicated adult tissues back to their totipotent embryological origins, from the specific functioning of an epithelial cell or cardiac tissue to the general capacity to create an entire organism found only in the earliest embryos. The birth of Dolly was the first time that a singular mammal, a particular sheep, could be reanimated as a new generation, a second life generated directly from the first.

To put it another way, Dolly demonstrated the capacity of oocytes to reactivate the embryological potential of all adult mammalian life and suggested that embryological life was a latent aspect of every human and animal tissue. Her existence suggested that any generation of mammals, including humans, could double or triple, or infinitely repeat their position in subsequent generations. Generational time had lost its sequential, successive character, and had instead become reiterative, restartable. Her existence also demonstrated that the singularity of mammalian being was no longer secure. While monozygotic twinning was a naturally occurring variation in mammalian reproduction, in which two or more siblings might share a genome, SCNT involves the production of twins in generations subsequent to each other, with the possibility that several different generations of the same creature could coexist in time. It suggested that the death of singular creatures was no longer a final termination point, because each singular creature could, potentially, rerun its development and life course through SCNT.

Dolly, and the development of the SCNT technique, hence threw many of the scientific and popular assumptions about biological time and mammalian life into disarray. Mammalian life includes human life, and the possibility that SCNT could be used for human reproduction precipitated a moral panic throughout the world. Human cloning was already a possibility richly developed in dystopian science fiction. The theme was well established in the twentieth-century public imagination around new reproductive technologies, as I explore in chapter 2 (Huxford 2000).

Public reception and the media framing of Dolly's birth revisited these dystopian tropes, raising the specter that, for example, the very wealthy might have themselves cloned to circumvent their own mortality, or that grieving parents might resurrect a dead child.[3] Government responses to the dislocation and moral panic precipitated by Dolly varied widely. In the United States, the announcement of Dolly produced a flurry of hastily drafted anticloning legislation, some concerned to ban all forms of SCNT, some focused on withholding federal funds from SCNT research, and some attempting to navigate through the condemnatory rhetoric to secure a research capacity for nonreproductive applications of SCNT (Gottweis, Salter, and Waldby 2009). In the UK, the existing history of well-regulated reproductive science and embryo research, combined with the fact that Dolly was a British "invention," created a space in which the more alarming possibilities could be contained, while research toward clinical applications could be explored.

In particular, the HFEA's consultation document *Cloning Issues in Reproduction, Science and Medicine* (Human Fertilisation and Embryology Authority 1998) made a crucial distinction between reproductive and what it termed "therapeutic" cloning. Reproductive cloning described the process used to create Dolly or any other entire organism, where the somatic cell of an adult is used as the nuclear material for a new birth. The document recommended a blanket ban on all human reproductive cloning, a ban enacted in legislation in many other jurisdictions, as states acted to contain the moral threat presented by SCNT. Reproductive cloning was antithetical to public good, the report argued, because it would treat the clone as a means to an end (the recreation of a dead child, the pursuit of personal immortality) rather than as an end in his or herself, and would pose potential, unknown health risk to the cloned person. A cloned child would have an unprecedented form of kinship with the "donor" parent, a situation that could involve psychological harm to both parent and child.

Therapeutic cloning, on the other hand, was discussed and recommended as a promising clinical application for the SCNT technique, combined with the then-new field of embryonic stem cell research. It would create not entire new organisms but rather histocompatible patient-specific tissues suitable for transplant. In this process, the nucleus from a patient's somatic cell, such as a skin cell, is introduced into an unfertilized oocyte from which the original genetic material has been removed. The oocyte is then used to produce a blastocyst (an early embryo) whose stem cells could be used to create tissue that would be compatible with that of the patient. Histocompatible tissue is highly desirable for many kinds of therapy because allogeneic tissues, those donated by another, always induce some degree of rejection by the patient's immune system. Organ recipients are dependent on powerful immunosuppressive medication to retain the organ. Moreover, embryonic stem cell lines present the possibility of endless supply; while donation rates for solid organs and blood products are rarely sufficient to meet ever-growing demand, stem cell tissues can, in theory, be multiplied and scaled up indefinitely. It also presented the possibility that degenerative conditions currently untreatable through donation, such as Parkinson's disease, could be addressed with pluripotent tissues that might be induced to engraft in the brain, or at other degenerated sites. Hence therapeutic cloning proffered a dramatic innovation in clinical treatments for conditions unaddressed by existing systems of tissue procurement.

The careful negotiation of this distinction between dystopian reproductive cloning and clinically beneficent therapeutic cloning, in the UK and then successively in several other jurisdictions, meant a way forward for human SCNT (Slabbert and Pepper 2015).[4] While most jurisdictions in the OECD had framed statutes banning human reproductive cloning, by the mid-2000s several had developed bodies of legislation and regulatory systems that facilitated some SCNT research for therapeutic applications. So in Australia, the Prohibition of Human Cloning and the Regulation of Human Embryo Research Amendment Act 2006 set out the conditions under which SCNT could be legally conducted, and set up a licensing system to approve particular laboratories. In the United Kingdom in 2006, the Human Fertilisation and Embryology Authority (HFEA) enabled egg-sharing arrangements to be extended for research oocyte donors, so that women seeking a reduction of their fertility treatment costs could provide a set proportion of their oocytes to stem cell research (Slabbert and Pepper 2015).

While the rhetorical stakes around SCNT were always high, the actual practice proved unattractive to all but a handful of laboratories around the world. Human SCNT presents a significant ethical and logistical problem. For biologists to develop the technical repertoire and precise protocols that might lead to successful creation of an SCNT cell line, the laboratory needs a steady, generous supply of fertile human oocytes. How to procure this supply was not evident. Two different strategies emerged in the first decade of this century. In the UK, building on the historical ethic of citizenship and mutual responsibility that underpins practices like blood donation (Waldby and Mitchell 2006), appeals were made to altruism. In 2005, Ian Wilmut, creator of Dolly the sheep, called for young British women to donate oocytes to assist with stem cell research into motor neuron disease. In an interview with the *Guardian*, Professor Wilmut said, "I have never doubted that women would donate if they thought we were helping people to have treatment. Our hope and belief is that women who have seen the devastating effect of this disease will be prepared to make such a donation" (Sample and Macleod 2005, n.p.).

Alongside these hypothetical young women were a more proximate group: women in IVF treatment. This patient group was the source of donation for human embryonic stem cell research. Patients undergoing IVF had proved themselves prepared to donate "spare" embryos, those not needed for their own reproductive aims, to laboratories carrying out stem cell research. This donation was altruistically framed—there were no incentives involved; they did not, at least in the UK and Australian systems, receive reduced treatment costs or compensation. It seemed to follow that this group might also be prepared to donate spare oocytes.

The alternative model derived from the commercial procurement practices of the U.S. fertility sector—the recruitment of young, nonpatient donors who provide oocytes for a fee. This model was profoundly compromised by the Hwang scandal in 2005. South Korean scientist Hwang Woo Suk and his team published two fraudulent papers in *Science* (in 2004 and 2005) falsely claiming to have created the world's first human SCNT cell lines. The fraud was eventually exposed, with dramatic consequences not only for Professor Hwang but also for the government. The South Korean government was intent on promoting Hwang as a national hero, so his laboratory received extensive support without scientific oversight. While the Ministry of Science formed a national Bioethics Advisory Committee in 2001, in response to stem cell controversy, its recommendations went largely ignored by the government. Hwang's SCNT research was later granted an exemption from statutory regulation by the 2005 Bioethics and Biosafety Act. The distribution of grants for stem cell research was based not on peer review but on government decisions. As a consequence, the exposure of the fraudulent research nearly brought down the government. Both the minister for science and the head of the BAC resigned (Gottweis, Salter, and Waldby 2009).

The Hwang scandal also galvanized and brought wider attention to the feminist critiques of stem cell research concerning the potentially exploitative nature of oocyte donation. Hwang and his team, in their attempt to create human SCNT cell lines, had procured 2,221 eggs from 121 women, most from brokers that normally sold Korean oocytes to Japanese fertility tourists. The rest were donated, including from two research assistants in Hwang's own laboratory team (Leem and Park 2008). When the research fraud scandal broke, the world's media were also alerted to an ethical issue that had gone relatively unremarked in the early 2000s debates about the status of embryonic life. That is, the dependence of SCNT and many other kinds of stem cell research (embryonic, hematopoietic, and fetal) on women's reproductive biology and the often onerous nature of the medical processes that precede donation. Feminist academics already researching the commercial transaction of oocytes and concerned about clinical risks and the inducement of women to provide eggs for money, have been working to bring attention to the ethical dangers presented by SCNT research (see, for example, Dodds 2003; Dickenson 2004), and this concern abruptly gained immense publicity and policy action.

The global reverberations of the Hwang scandal effectively placed a moratorium on frank payment for research oocytes, even in those jurisdictions like California where reproductive oocytes markets had operated since the 1980s. At the same time, few women have proved willing to give oocytes for SCNT research gratuitously. For several years after the Hwang scandal, it seemed that there was no viable, ethically defensible procurement model for research oocytes. More recently, however, a handful of laboratories have found ways to renew paid procurement, and these have been the loci of recent success in creating human SCNT lines. In the United States, the procurement systems have developed around a labor model, one that closely maps the historical dynamics that Melinda Cooper and I explored in our book *Clinical Labor* (Cooper and Waldby 2014).

In what follows, I briefly go back to the fieldwork with former Australian IVF patients that I drew on in chapter 3, as well as considering the reasoning about time, work, and research donation that emerged from an additional cohort of informants: young, well-educated Australian women without direct experience of IVF. These two cohorts are relevant to an understanding of research donation because they each represent a possible source of such donation: women already in treatment, and young, nonpatient women at peak fertility who might be recruited to provide research oocytes. I then return to the particular regulatory developments in the United States that have facilitated the creation of a professionalized provider panel for research oocytes.

Time, Labor, Payment

In vitro fertilization patients have proved willing to donate embryos to stem cell research as gifts to blue-sky research, so it seems plausible that patients might also be prepared to donate oocytes. My analysis in chapter 3 of responses from former IVF patients, however, showed that the technical features of oocytes, their lack of affordance points, their singularity and intractability, their opacity to ranking and sorting, rendered women going through IVF very unwilling to provide their oocytes to others. This opacity is particularly difficult for SCNT donation, because oocytes must be diverted from the reproductive path onto the research path *prior to fertilization*. The SCNT process utilizes the fertilization mechanisms of the oocyte specifically, and indeed these mechanisms are necessary for the technique to work at all. These oocytes can be used only once, and used entirely, so they must be diverted *either* into reproductive or research pathways, in a zero-sum fashion.

Several women from the former patient group stated that they had no objection to donating eggs that failed to fertilize. While eggs that fail to fertilize have some technical value for laboratories, allowing researchers to optimize some techniques, they cannot be used for actual SCNT attempts. Once this necessity was explained to the interviewees, they almost without exception withdrew their preparedness to give. Nadia was bleakly amused by the expectation that any woman in IVF would give potentially fertile eggs to research. "[Laughs.] They need the best ones! Oh, then, no! How can I give them . . . that's the problem. What I thought, if they didn't want the best ones, then I can ask the scientists, 'Can I keep the best ones, and you keep the others!' [Laughs.] Oh, that's hard" (Nadia, ex-IVF patient, late twenties, married, student, one child).

Another significant constraint on donation is related to the life course of IVF patients. Generally speaking, women and couples present to IVF clinics in the woman's mid- to late thirties or early forties, after several years of conception attempts. This history might involve repeated miscarriage, dealing with clinical conditions like endometriosis or polycystic ovary syndrome, or simply repeated disappointments, as conception remains elusive. Hence IVF patients understand their treatment as their last chance to form a family before their reproductive capacities are entirely extinguished. Most of the women interviewed stated that, if they were younger and their fertility were abundant, they would at least consider research donation, and some stated they would certainly donate. Sarah expressed this preparedness in the following terms.

> [In] an IVF cycle, you're doing it purely and simply to have a baby. If I was in a position where I knew I had lots of eggs—and usually it's girls in their twenties that have plenty to offer and those that have maybe already had children—if I was in that circumstance, then I would definitely consider it. I'd *want* to be able to share my fertility with others or, you know, that benefit . . . others. So I wouldn't have an issue with donating in that circumstance but I am forty now, or I will be in December and I'm not really very fertile anymore! (Sarah, ex-IVF patient, late thirties, accountant, married, one child)

This is a succinct expression of the conflict for fertility patients when faced with an invitation to donate for research. In a hypothetical situation of abundance, Sarah would like to share her fertility, make it available for others, including those who might benefit from SCNT research. As an IVF patient, however, she is faced with the oocyte deficit that is almost always concomitant with fertility treatment. In her response, we see the deeply felt sense that fertility is a capacity that *should* be devoted to the creation of children, to the succession of generational time and the couples' desire for family life and continuity. If the fertility of oocytes could also be devoted to the creation of SCNT cell lines, and eventually to therapies, the women perceived this as a residual quality, one that they might consider under certain circumstances but that did not exercise large claims on them.

So among former patient interviewees, there was a broad consensus that women in fertility treatment should not be asked to donate for research. The request was framed as inappropriate and unethical, involving exactly those women least able to afford a response. When we turn to the focus groups, involving young nonpatient women, we get a somewhat different set of concerns. First, the possibility of donation *after* the completion of family was repeatedly considered by the focus group participants. Their willingness to entertain the idea of altruistic research donation emphasizes the significance of life course trajectories in these considerations. All were under thirty years old, and none had children at the time. Almost all were undergraduate or postgraduate students, and so the process of family formation was somewhat hypothetical and held off until some point in the future. Research donation could be entertained as an additional element to these hypothetical scenarios, something to be undertaken after the goals of childbirth are achieved.

> If I had three kids, I think I could donate all my eggs to research, because I'd be sure I don't want any other children. (Martha, late twenties, doctoral student)

> I think, . . . Why would I want to let good eggs go to waste? The chances are that I've got more stored . . . and these are really good eggs that people could use but I don't know. I think, in another sense, I'd probably rather donate *after* I had a kid, if I was planning on having a kid, just because it's like, . . . What do I need the rest for? (Eveline, early twenties, undergraduate student)

The young women were prepared to locate a point in their life course where they could afford to give oocytes to research, a point at which they had established their own families and could be certain they did not need their remaining fertility. Some stated a preference for research over reproductive donation. They were worried that reproductive donation would bring with it ethical and maternal concerns about the life of their genetic child, whom they could not care for, while research donation did not involve specific responsibilities.

> I'd probably feel differently about donating eggs for research as opposed to donating eggs for reproduction. Strangely enough, I think I'd feel happy about donating eggs for research . . . because I just personally don't want to have a half-child out there and not know them. (Albertine, mid-twenties, undergraduate student)

At the same time, the young women stated clearly that their preparedness to donate would depend on specific therapeutic applications of their tissue.

I think it would have to be a very good cause, though. So, say—I don't know, if I knew someone, or if my partner had a spinal injury, and the possibility of me donating my eggs after I'd had children would possibly find a cure for *him*, then yes, of course I'd do it, but it has to be a very good cause or a very personal cause, as opposed to just *any* old research. (Celeste, mid-twenties, undergraduate student)

Several of the young women mentioned specific conditions they would consider appropriate for research donation, as Celeste does above, but they also tied treatments to particular friends or relatives who suffer from such conditions. That is, they were prepared to consider donation to help a particular person, and by extension others with the same condition.

On face value, then, it appears as though young, educated women, insofar as the focus groups and interviews could be considered representative, would be potential altruistic oocyte donors for SCNT research, if the research were sufficiently applied and had a proximate therapeutic application. As the focus group discussions and interviews evolved, however, it became evident that other considerations come into play. In particular, the time commitment associated with oocyte donation featured as a significant constraint on willingness to donate altruistically. The participants repeatedly described oocyte donation as difficult because of the time-consuming procedures. The extended duration of donation displaced other possible uses of the donor's time:

If circumstances were different, I would look at [donating oocytes] differently. And not working . . . [laughs]. You know, it's such a difficult thing to manage. For eight weeks, you have to be regimented that at twelve-hourly intervals you're doing a medication thing. And it extremely affects your mood: you can't work and manage the drugs and manage a family life. (Nadia, ex-IVF patient, late twenties, married, student, one child)

Nadia and many other participants from all cohorts pointed out that the time demands of oocyte donation displaced other forms of *productive* time, particular the time necessary to earn an income. Hence, the time involved in producing oocytes takes on an implied equivalence with work, that is, with *paid* time. Respondents repeatedly argued that compensation should be calculated according to this equivalence.

I think compensation should be given according to the amount of time that's involved, [which] . . . would be two to three weeks. . . . I think it would probably make people more prepared to do it, if they don't have to combine it with the stresses of work . . . if it takes someone two weeks to go through an IVF process, or sixteen days or whatever, that they be given that time off work on full pay. (Philippa, ex-IVF patient, late forties, media producer, de facto relationship, one child)

Among the young nonpatient group, there was also a vivid sense of the potential *commercial* value of biomedical research. They made a marked distinction between personal acts of reproductive or research donation to a loved one, and the more anonymous provision of biological material to a research facility. Perhaps reflecting their experience with the contemporary commercialized university, they regarded medical research as a business, and hence an appropriate location for some form of monetary transaction. As Eveline puts it,

I have less of an issue with [payment for] research than for reproduction. . . . Like, for research, it seems more like they should pay me for it, because you pay when you do research. You pay for things. You pay for materials, you pay study subjects to do focus groups with you . . . ! [Laughs.] So it just seems more fitting for there to be payment for research than it does for there to be payment for [reproduction]. (Eveline, early twenties, undergraduate student)

The purpose of research is not the creation of a child, but the creation of knowledge. The young women were aware of the commercial potential of biomedical discovery and considered that altruistic donation of materials that could give rise to profitable knowledge and patent would be inherently unfair.

I'd want them to pay me! [Laughs.] If I thought that some profit was going to come of it in the end, I would at least want something more than reimbursed travel, I guess. (Rosanne, mid-twenties, undergraduate student)

I would have a real problem with donating eggs that would then be used to create technology that was then patented and charged prohibitive prices for. (Francine, mid-twenties, undergraduate student)

The young women felt entitled to some equity in potentially profitable research, and thought that compensation rates should reflect this. *The exchange value of oocytes is derived not only from time equivalence but also from commercial conditions and the patentability of research tissues.* At the same time, this group was aware of the issue of undue inducement, and the ethical problems raised by higher rates of compensation that bled over into frank payment. They expressed concerns regarding the power of money to attract impoverished or simply opportunistic donors, who might overlook the dangers of participation or be unconcerned about the public good aspects of the research itself. Donna expresses this paradox precisely:

> I agree that it's a concern that women who wouldn't otherwise donate eggs would do so for financial reasons. . . . They may sign the consent forms without . . . acknowledging or being able to understand or incorporate the actual risks because they're just looking at the money because they're in financial distress. But on the other hand, I don't see why women shouldn't be paid to go through a surgical process and to go through and basically contribute to scientific research. . . . On a bit of a cynical note, if a drug company or a medical research company does come up with a solution that's going to cure Alzheimer's or whatever, . . . the pharmaceutical company is going to recuperate significantly more revenue than it cost to develop the research, so why should they [the donors] get a free ride? (Donna, early twenties, undergraduate student)

An expectation of equity in the context of commercial medical research is in something of a conflict with the community ethics of donation. A significant proportion of the ex-fertility patients (thirteen out of twenty) also considered that young women should be paid for research donation, and their reasons were for the most part similar to those of the young women—that commercially driven, profitable research organizations should be obliged to pay tissue providers accordingly.

Research Payment and Clinical Labor

In summary, the former patients and nonpatient women expressed a considerable degree of consensus about oocyte procurement for SCNT research. This consensus suggests a professionalization process around

SCNT oocyte provision, one somewhat similar to the reproductive sector in the United States, where young women are extensively screened for both particular genetic and social qualities to become part of a panel providing sometimes several cycles in return for fees (Almeling 2011). Another way to put this is that the study participants considered that research oocyte provision should move toward what I term a "clinical labor model," one in which the economic value of the transaction is more transparent, and women have a more clearly contractual status as providers of an in vivo service (Cooper and Waldby 2014). In this framework, oocyte providers are recognized and treated explicitly as workers located inside the value chain of the life sciences, rather than as donors who give from the social sphere to research institutions in an ethic of civil generosity.

If we look at the landscape of SCNT research since the Hwang scandal, we indeed see an incremental yet steady shift toward a regularized clinical labor model. As I noted above, the frank payment for research oocytes was ethically vexed by the Hwang scandal in the first decade of the twenty-first century, even in jurisdictions that had long tolerated reproductive oocyte transactions, and for a few years it appeared that the scandal had made any attempt to transact research oocytes ethically indefensible. This dynamic is most evident in California, one of the U.S. states with a well-developed entrepreneurial *reproductive* oocyte market, where women who meet stringent physical, social, and educational standards are paid US$7,000 to US$10,000 per cycle to provide eggs to fertility patients. California is also the location of the world's most lavish publicly funded stem cell research facility, the California Institute for Regenerative Medicine (CIRM), created in 2006 through Proposition 71 to secure the state's position as a global leader in the field.

In the process of California's creating the CIRM and framing state legislation to support its work, an extensive network of feminist, civil, and health activists mobilized around the issue of payment for research oocytes. Charis Thompson notes that several U.S. controversies regarding biological tissue were also uppermost in activists minds at the time, in addition to the Hwang scandal—she lists the HeLa controversy, in which an African American woman, Henrietta Lacks, had provided cervical cancer cells to research without informed consent in the 1950s, cells that were used to create the first immortalized cell line; the use of Havasupai blood samples without consent, brought to suit in 2008; and the use of infant blood samples without consent in Texas (Thompson 2013). The

Pro Choice Alliance for Responsible Research argued for a moratorium on payment for *research* donation, citing the risks and opportunities for coercion (Benjamin 2013), despite the absence of such demands in relation to reproductive donation over the twenty-five years that fertility clinics had been using payment. Thompson argues that the difference in activists' approach to research versus reproductive oocyte provision arose from

> the public nature of stem cell research versus the private nature of assisted reproductive technologies (ARTS), the fact that in ARTS the eggs stay within the context of reproductive intent whereas they exit it for stem cell research, and the stratified nature of egg donation for ARTS. Needing the popular vote, being funded with taxpayer money, and being under the strict ethical and licensing regimes of scientific research all made egg donation for stem cell research subject to much more public scrutiny and oversight than ARTS, which had always managed in the United States to work largely out of the public eye. (Thompson 2013, 105–106)

The activist position was eventually encoded in the 2006 California legislation The Reproductive Health and Research Bill (SB1260), which states that "no payment in excess of the amount of reimbursement of direct expenses incurred as a result of the procedure shall be made to any subject to encourage her to produce human oocytes for the purposes of medical research."[5]

The effect of this strict reimbursement model *operating alongside a transactional reproductive market* is that several laboratories in California that had embarked on SCNT research abandoned the field by 2012, as they were unable to secure a supply of fertile oocytes. In fieldwork carried out in 2010, Braun and Schultz identified two California institutes still involved in the area: ISCO Oceanside, which was planning to launch an egg-sharing scheme, where women would receive subsidized fertility treatment in exchange for donating a proportion of their oocyte for research; and Stemagen, who had brokered a complex reallocation system. The laboratory worked with an egg brokerage company and a fertility clinic to divert eggs sold for reproductive purposes into SCNT research. Both the provider and the recipients had to consent to this diversion. This reallocation model effectively free rides on the transactional market for reproductive oocytes yet complies with the regulations insofar as there was no additional payment at the point of diversion (Braun and Schultz

2012). The complexity of this approach, however, eventually led the laboratory to close its SCNT program, and no SCNT work was in progress in California by 2014, when I carried out fieldwork there (interview Alan Trounson 2014).

In Europe, a similar winnowing process had reduced the number of laboratories involved in SCNT work from six in 2007 to three in 2010. The laboratories that abandoned the research all cited the difficulty of securing oocyte supply and the impracticality of reliance on IVF patients. In each case they moved to iPSC work instead. The three remaining laboratories, two in Spain, and one in the UK, had each brokered compromises between anticommercialization statutes that prohibited payment and methods of compensating oocyte providers. The Spanish laboratories each set up a reallocation system similar to Stemagen's, diverting oocytes from highly compensated reproductive providers to research, while the Herbert Laboratory at Newcastle on Tyne is funded by the Medical Research Council to subsidize IVF treatment for women who agree to give a proportion of their eggs to research. While this approach is modeled on the long-standing UK egg-sharing model for reproductive donation, it nevertheless ties the laboratory to oocytes from women who themselves generally have compromised fertility (Braun and Schultz 2012).

By 2016, two laboratories in the United States, one in New York and the other in Oregon, had developed a professionalized provider panel of young, nonpatient women paid a fee for research oocytes. Notably, in neither state was there a protracted public-funding battle as in California, even though New York State had embarked on a significant publicly funded process for stem cell research in 2007, committing US$600 million over eleven years. The governing council, the Empire State Stem Cell Board, undertook a two-year deliberative process through its ethics committee to formulate defensible guidelines for payment that model phase one clinical trial participation. Their guidelines mandate a US$10,000 fee for research oocytes, funded from the state's public research budget. This approach effectively meets the U.S. market rate for reproductive oocytes (Levine 2010) and makes New York the first state in the world to "affirmatively allow" *payment*, rather than compensation, for research oocytes (Foohey 2010; NYSTEM Strategic Planning Coordinating Committee 2015). Payment, however, is for time and the onerous nature of the process. It is not, according to the guidelines, an amount of money paid for the oocytes themselves (Roxland 2012, 405). Participants are also

screened, monitored, and treated with nonaggressive hormone stimulation, and the laboratory grant holders are responsible for medical follow-
up and costs in the case of clinical problems from the donation process
(Roxland 2012, 400).

The Egli Laboratory at the New York Stem Cell Foundation used this
procurement route to create a provider panel of nonpatient women
between twenty-one and thirty-four years old, who were recruited from
among participants in the reproductive oocyte donation program of a New
York fertility clinic. The women were approached about research donation only after they had been screened and approved for reproductive
donation. Consistent with the social profile of approved reproductive
providers, the women were well educated, with at minimum a college
degree. The first SCNT study developed from this panel involved the creation of triploid SCNT blastocysts (with both the oocyte nucleus and an
introduced somatic cell nucleus) and embryonic stem cell lines in 2011
(Noggle et al. 2011). This study enrolled sixteen women, who together
provided 270 mature oocytes for an US$8,000 fee per cycle, the same
amount they would have earned for reproductive provision. The study,
while a technical advance in the science in some respects, was not received as a therapeutically useful one, because no patient-specific lines
could be derived from triploid blastocysts.

The Egli Laboratory then went on to successfully create patient-
specific SCNT lines (Yamada et al. 2014), but the first group to establish
human SCNT lines was based in Oregon and led by Shoukhrat Mitalipov
(Tachibana et al. 2013). This laboratory too had access to paid oocyte providers, through their relationship with a fertility clinic. Like the Egli Lab,
they avoided the politicization evident in California, in part because they
avoided publicity until they had reportable success, and in part because
they are a standalone clinical facility. The framing of procurement as payment for time mirrored that of the New York guidelines, and of the ASRM
sectoral guidelines as well. Oregon, like many other U.S. states, does not
directly regulate oocyte procurement for fertility or research purposes,
so the clinic could frame its own approach in harmonization with the
emerging business model articulated by the New York Stem Cell Board
(Ikemoto 2014, 7).

At the same time, the Oregon group could build its ethical argument
on a different basis than that of the New York researchers and most other

groups. The team developed much of its technical repertoire through experimentation on rhesus macaque oocytes, and several members were at the forefront of primate reproductive biology research (Trounson and DeWitt 2013). Hence, they were not dependent on extensive human oocyte procurement to refine their techniques. Once they moved to human SCNT work, their derivation process was notably efficient, in that six lines were created from oocytes provided by only three donors. They identified several procedures necessary to secure SCNT cell lines, including alteration to the stimulation protocols for the oocyte providers, rather than a simple adaptation of protocols used for reproductive provision. The researchers state in their published results, "Clearly, further studies addressing gonadotropin dosage and pituitary suppression regimens should be evaluated in the context of recovering human oocytes suitable for SCNT" (Tachibana et al. 2013, 1235) and that better, more specific screening tests were needed to identify women with optimal oocyte quality for SCNT research. These conclusions point toward the establishment of dedicated oocyte procurement systems for SCNT work, rather than one modeled on fertility clinic protocols.

Taken together, these two experimental sites suggest that only laboratories that can identify a specific, virtually professionalized cohort of oocyte providers and pay fees sufficient to attract them away from reproductive donation will be able to sustain an SCNT program. As SCNT becomes a more routine procedure, and as the value of comparative work with iPSCs is probed, oocyte providers could plausibly be integrated more explicitly into the productive infrastructure of biological innovation. That they are not positioned as *vendors*, selling the biological matériel itself, but as providers of a service is striking. While this framing avoids actual or potential anticommercialization statutes around the sale of body parts, it also tips the status of the women toward an explicit clinical labor model, where they are paid for time, risk, and expertise, as collaborators in a research program, rather than as donors who give from the social sphere to research institutions in an ethic of civil, feminine generosity (Cooper and Waldby 2014). This professionalization of research donation follows a similar trajectory as the that of the Californian egg bank donors described in chapter 5. In each case the potential recipients are remote, and the egg providers sell services to a biomedical institute rather than give a gift of fertility or regenerative potential to another.

Mitochondrial Transplantation

While SCNT research is speculative at best, focused on discovery and laboratory development, and a long way from applications, oocytes have recently acquired a much more proximate clinical value. In February 2015,
the British House of Commons and the House of Lords voted to permit
a technique termed "mitochondrial replacement," a way for women with
inherited disorders in their mitochondrial DNA to conceive a child free
from those diseases (Kmietowicz 2015). The vote created an amendment
to the Human Fertilization and Embryology Act (1990, amended 2008),
which would allow the creation of embryos using the enucleated egg of
a donor and the fertilized zygotic pronuclei of the intending parents.
As the press headlines dutifully announced, the embryo would be the
creation of three people, or more sensationally, a "three parent embryo"
(Connor 2015), combining the nuclear DNA of the parents proper and the
healthy mitochondrial DNA of the egg donor. While women with mitochondrial disorders in their family had until this point relied on IVF and
the usual vagaries of oocyte donation, or on highly variable success with
preimplantation genetic diagnosis (PGD) to identify an embryo with a low
burden of mutated mDNA, they could now look forward to conceiving a
healthy child that would count as genetically their own, if genetic identity
is limited to nuclear DNA. This limit, however, is tendentious.

Mitochondria form part of the genetic material transmitted by the
oocyte, with their origins in very early evolution of multicellular eukaryotic life. In a symbiotic relationship, the mitochondria and the nuclear
DNA in the cell effectively form the basic structure of all multicellular life.
Unlike nuclear DNA, however, which recombines and mutates in sexual
reproduction, mDNA does not routinely recombine, so that its conforma-
tion remains very stable over time (Stewart and Chinnery 2015). Mitochondrial genes pass down the maternal line in almost identical form
over many generations, as the mDNA material in the oocyte divides
among the embryonic cells during early development and becomes part
of each cell in the offspring. Cells contain multiple copies of mDNA,
ranging from a few hundred in sperm to thousands in oocytes, and this
distribution contributes to the complexity and unpredictability of mutations, which may vary in concentration between the same tissues in an
organ and the same organs in an individual. Extended kinship networks

through the maternal line will share identical mitochondrial DNA, and inheritance is so stable over time that it is used by population geneticists and physical anthropologists to track the deep history of human migration and diffusion (Stewart and Chinnery 2015).[6]

Because mitochondria are involved in cell metabolism and energy production, mitochondrial disorders disable organs with high energy requirements, particularly neurological, hepatic, and cardiac tissues. This feature, combined with the variable distribution of mutations, creates the characteristic heterogeneity of clinical symptoms. They manifest in a broad and often grave range of conditions, including stroke, dementia, epilepsy, organ failure, diabetes, and premature death. Asymptomatic mothers may conceive children with severe disease, and symptoms may only emerge late in life. An estimated one in four thousand to five thousand people are affected by mitochondrial disease (Cree and Loi 2015), although given the extreme heterogeneity of the symptoms, it is also thought to be underdiagnosed and underreported (Nuffield Council on Bioethics 2012). Treatment for mitochondrial disease is primarily organized through diagnostic testing and symptom management. In Britain the NHS has established a specialized clinic at Newcastle University that brings together diagnostic, research, and multidisciplinary medical expertise to provide comprehensive care for severely affected patients. The clinic director explained to me the reasoning behind the clinic's interest in reproductive techniques:

> So, if you look at the ethos of our Centre, it's really about: how can we improve the lives of patients with mitochondrial disease? . . . Improving diagnosis improves their lives. . . . We can then tailor the treatment optimally, and . . . we've established the first clinical guidelines for patients with mitochondrial disease, with streamline testing. We, as I say, provide a national service, so we really are focused . . . looking for new drugs, running clinical trials . . . all the sort of things that we would want to do. So, one of the things that's obvious . . . was: we've got to get better at making genetic diagnosis, because in a fatal disease, providing reproductive choice is the *only* option. . . . I think some of the next generation of sequencing technique[s] will allow us to get much better at doing that with nuclear gene disorders, but the mitochondrial gene that was sequenced in 1981—the first mutations

were discovered in 1988. We've known about those mutations for years. And what became quite clear to us, and to those of us looking after the patients, is that we need to do better about giving reproductive advice and, in fairness, reproductive choice to women who carry these mutations.

Because mitochondrial disorders are not curable, the only definitive way to address the condition is to prevent the conception of children who will inherit the disorders. Unlike some other genetic conditions, mDNA disorders are not readily identified through PGD, in which a cell is removed from a developing embryo for testing. Preimplantation genetic diagnosis is widely used to select embryos free of readily diagnosable genetic conditions like Huntington chorea or cystic fibrosis (Lu et al. 2016), but the severity of mDNA mutations are often difficult to assess in the embryo, and PGD is of no assistance in cases of homoplasmy, which affects all embryos (Hellebrekers et al. 2012). Hence, the only method that guarantees that mDNA conditions will not be inherited is to disrupt the line of maternal mitochondrial descent. At this point, oocyte donation and the technique of mitochondrial transplantation come into play.

Mitochondrial transplantation can be performed in two ways—pronuclear transfer and maternal spindle transfer. In the first, the pronuclei (the nuclear DNA from sperm and egg of the intending parents) found in the one-day-old single-cell-fertilized human embryo (zygote) are removed, leaving behind the mother's cytoplasm and the mitochondria. They are then transplanted into a donor oocyte that has been enucleated, but which contains the healthy mitochondria of the donor. The zygote then develops normally into a blastocyst, embryo, fetus, and infant, and each of its cells will contain both the parental nuclear DNA and the donor mDNA. In the second, the spindle from the unfertilized oocyte of a woman with mDNA disease in her family is transferred to an enucleated donor oocyte (Amato et al. 2014). While the procedure has been approved in principle in the UK, to date only one child has been born through this technique, performed in Mexico by a U.S. clinical team who relocated to avoid U.S. prohibitions (Hamzelou 2016). The Newcastle Centre is mounting a five-year trial of the treatment, being conducted 2017–2022.

Mitochondrial Identity and Germ Line Modification

The treatment is intended to give women with mitochondrial disease in their family the possibility to conceive a child who is genetically their own yet free of mDNA disorders. The Nuffield Council report on the practice, commissioned to provide ethical guidance and evaluation, states: "New variations of IVF techniques are being developed that aim to replace damaged mitochondria by using part of a donated egg from a healthy individual. The intention is to allow women carrying disorders of mitochondrial DNA the chance to have healthy children that are genetically related to them, but born free of those disorders. Such techniques are not currently permitted for treatment use under UK legislation" (Nuffield Council on Bioethics 2012, xv). The last sentence refers to the prohibition against genetic modification, or "germ line modification," as it is sometimes termed, under the HFE Act (1990, 2008), in force until the recent modification described earlier in this chapter. This legislation explicitly bundled nuclear and mitochondrial DNA as substances that could not be legally modified in the embryo. Section 3ZA "permitted eggs, permitted sperm and permitted embryos" explicitly excludes eggs and embryos "whose nuclear or mitochondrial DNA has . . . been altered."[7] This prohibition complies with international norms that guard against germ line modification, encoded in the UN *Universal Declaration on the Human Genome and Human Rights* (UNESCO 1997) and most recently articulated by the moratorium on human gene editing declared in December 2015 by the National Academy of Sciences of the United States, the Institute of Medicine, the Chinese Academy of Sciences, and the Royal Society of London. The moratorium statement argues that human germ line editing in embryos poses extensive clinical risk for any child born as a result, but more importantly, it poses risks to future generations, because any modification would be inherited. The technique raises

> the obligation to consider implications for both the individual and the future generations who will carry the genetic alterations; . . . the fact that, once introduced into the human population, genetic alterations would be difficult to remove and would not remain within any single community or country; . . . the possibility that permanent genetic "enhancements" to subsets of the population could exacerbate social inequities or be used coercively; and . . . the moral and ethical

considerations in purposefully altering human evolution using this technology.[8]

Nevertheless, the HFE Act goes on specifically to note a possible exception to its prohibited eggs and embryos in cases of "a prescribed process designed to prevent the transmission of serious mitochondrial disease." This caveat formed the basis for the parliamentary ruling I describe earlier in this chapter.

So in summary, following the logic of the HFE Act and the more recent parliamentary ruling, mDNA transplantation is constituted as an exception to a more general norm that prohibits inheritable modification. It is deemed legitimate because it enables women with mDNA disorders to have a genetically related child and prevent further transmission of serious mitochondrial disease.

This logic suggests a quite particular understanding of genetic relatedness, however, and of the significance of the mitochondria in the capacities of the oocyte. In the following section I consider the relationship between how mitochondrial DNA is understood and how a mitochondrial donor is recognized in the UK regulatory framework. I discuss in chapter 4 how particular understandings of genetics and gestation informed the sense of entitlement women felt toward their donor-conceived children, and toward the donor herself. The more convinced they were that kinship is created by nuclear DNA, the more they felt that the child was not properly "theirs." Rather they felt the egg donor was the true mother. We can see a similar, synecdochal relationship between the figuration of mitochondria, nuclear DNA, donor, recipient, and child in the key documents informing the debate and regulation of the field. Succinctly put, the more instrumental the understanding of mDNA, the less recognition is afforded the donor. In what follows I explore this synecdoche in detail.

The Mitochondrial Gift

One of the key regulatory problems thrown up by mDNA donation is the status of the donor. Reproductive egg donors in the UK, Australia, and several other countries are legally required to register their identities and to accept that any donor-conceived children will have access to this information once they turn eighteen. The rationale for registries relates to the understanding, derived historically from the sphere of adoption, that children have a right to knowledge of their biological parents if these are not the same persons as their social parents. While donors have no duty of care or obligation to the child, registration nevertheless recognizes the donor's status in a certain way, enshrining the relationship and documenting it through time as a significant contribution to the life of the child. In chapter 3 Australian reproductive donors indeed felt a sense of contribution and responsibility for the child conceived with their eggs, to the extent that they felt it was incumbent on them to assess the parental capacities of the recipients to decide whether they would be responsible parents. For the women I interviewed who traveled overseas for donation, this recognition was unwelcome, something to be evaded if possible, because it threw too much doubt on their own sense of maternal claim. Here we can see that particular understandings of egg donation and genetic relatedness are bound up with complex structures of feeling about the child, family formation, and how donors are figured.

Mitochondrial donation could, potentially, be classified in a similar way to reproductive donation. As Erica Haimes and Ken Taylor note, mitochondrial donation involves, after all, the provision of entire oocytes, rather than isolated mitochondrial tissue (Haimes and Taylor 2015). The process of donation is precisely the same as I describe in chapter 3 for reproductive oocytes; it involves extensive testing, stimulation regimes, clinic visits, ultrasound scans, and surgical egg retrieval. For any donor, the process is as demanding, time critical, and risky as it is for reproductive oocyte provision, and the oocytes themselves are as profoundly implicated in the creation of the pregnancy. As totipotent tissue, they necessarily direct the unfolding of the nuclear DNA and orchestrate the establishment of the embryo and the gestational conditions needed to constitute the child. The popular media coverage of mDNA therapy recognizes this contribution in its locution "three parent embryos" and three-parent babies, terms featured in headlines reporting on the UK parliamentary decision.[9]

Nevertheless, the terminology of "mitochondrial donation" suggests a far more modest, limited contribution from the donor. Haimes and Taylor observe that, in pronuclear transfer, the nuclear DNA material of the intending parents is transferred into the oocyte, while the terminology "mitochondrial donation" rather suggests the opposite, that the mDNA itself is transferred to the parents:

The term "mitochondrial donation" . . . implies that the egg provider contributes only mitochondria; however, her "host" egg contains not only mitochondria but also all the other cellular structures and chemicals required by the intending parents' nuclear DNA to direct the egg to develop into an embryo. Therefore, in the therapeutic applications, not only will the transfer of material be in the opposite direction to that usually implied, but also the contribution of the volunteer's host egg will be much more extensive than usually acknowledged. (Haimes and Taylor 2015, 6)

Haimes and Taylor's point is that the choice of term in the regulatory framing of the practice actively minimizes the contribution of the donor. If we scrutinize the key regulatory documents, they evince a strong concern to demonstrate that mitochondrial donors are *not* reproductive donors. In the guidance provided by the Human Fertilisation and Embryology Authority to the government on mitochondrial donation, and in the Nuffield Council's report on ethical and regulatory issues, both bodies argue *against* a recognition of the reproductive contribution of the donor. The HFEA advises that, "Mitochondria donors should have a similar status to that of tissue donors. Children born of mitochondria replacement should not have a right to access identifying information about the donor when they reach the age of 18" (Human Fertilisation and Embryology Authority 2013, 5). While the Nuffield Council reaches the same conclusion: "The donor of mitochondria should not have the same status in regulation as a reproductive egg or embryo donor in all aspects. As part of this, we do not believe mitochondrial donors should be mandatorily required to be identifiable to the adults born from their donation" (Nuffield Council on Bioethics 2012, xvi). These recommendations rest in turn on particular kinds of reasoning about the meaning and status of mitochondria, and the relative weight given to different kinds of genetic material in constituting the flow of generational time and family continuity. This weighting is driven largely, I would argue, by the social intentions inscribed in the therapeutic technique. Mitochondrial donation is described as giving parents with mDNA disorders in their family the opportunity to conceive a child who is genetically related to both the intending mother and the intending father. It is meant *precisely to displace the reliance on a reproductive egg donor*, which has been the most common treatment option up until this point. The displacement is notional, in the sense that mDNA therapy will be just as reliant on the availability of oocyte donors as is straightforward reproductive donation. Any such donation, however, will be framed as the gift of purely instrumental qualities, rather than the gift of self-identity that so troubles some egg recipients.

The pronuclear transfer technique dramatizes this intention in its meticulous manipulation of the sequence of conception. Each parental nuclear genome is captured at the singular moment when they are collocated together; yet the maternal oocyte, with its faulty mitochondria, has not yet begun to orchestrate the embryo. The pronuclei are isolated and transferred over to the donor oocyte, where their recombination can proceed accordingly. Here we can see that the donor oocyte is treated as an instrument dedicated to the sanctified expression of the couples' nuclear DNA. The biological asymmetry between the spermatic and oocytic contribution to the embryo, which I outline in chapter 1, is here effaced in the sense that the contribution of the intending parents is symmetrical—both contribute nuclear DNA—and nuclear DNA is figured as the material that transmits identity proper. Hence mDNA donor-conceived children are not the offspring of three parents because the third actor, the donor, does not partake in the creation of true identity. The reasoning here is well expressed by the British Medical Association's submission to the Nuffield Council inquiry:

> The child will be the child of the intended parents whose nuclear DNA is used to produce the embryo from which the child has developed. The donor of the mitochondrial DNA should not be considered in the same way as an egg donor since her contribution is to provide an energy source for the cells only. Although there is still much that is unknown about the role of mitochondrial DNA, the scientific consensus is that it does not have any influence on the characteristics of the child. The reason children born following donor conception require information about the donor is because the information relates to them as a person, and the donor's genes have contributed to that person's physical appearance and personal characteristics. The same does not apply to mitochondrial DNA (cited in Nuffield Council on Bioethics 2012, 74).

The notion that mDNA has a strictly instrumental, impersonal action for the person is repeatedly expressed in the key documents though the idea of batteries. The Nuffield report states, for example, "Enzymes in mitochondria convert the nutrients received from food into cellular energy. This is essential to the functioning of cells in the human body. Mitochondria have been described as 'the powerhouse of the cell,' and have sometimes been referred to as the 'batteries in a cell,' due to their generation of energy" (Nuffield Council on Bioethics 2012, 18).

The Lily Foundation, a patient organization for mDNA conditions, uses the battery locution in its description of mitochondrial donation, which is "like replacing the batteries in a toy—the toy remains exactly the same, it just has the power to work properly."[10] And the Wellcome Trust Centre for Mitochondrial Research has a YouTube presentation on its website titled "Healing Broken Batteries."[11]

Here we can see that, if mitochondria are simply batteries to drive the mechanisms of the cells, they are both quite impersonal mechanical entities and readily replaced. Like batteries proper they can simply be changed, *indeed they are designed to be changed*, and if changed they do not affect the nature of the mechanism they drive or the child conceived through the therapy. Patients with mDNA disorders were involved in the HFEA consultation, and their transcribed understandings expressed this idea of mitochondria as uninvolved and detachable: "They stressed that mitochondrial DNA is only involved in energy production and that a child's sense of self would be derived from his/her nuclear DNA which would still be inherited from the parents. *'Everything that makes you "you" and that makes your child "your child" is not touched.'* Participant F" (Sheikh 2013, 13). So mitochondrial transplantation is a neutral technique that does not shape the identity of the child, if mitochondria are discrete exchangeable elements in the cell, and if identity proper is transmitted through nuclear DNA. We can discern here a narrow understanding of mitochondria and of mDNA therapy, which shores up the social intent of the technique and positions donors as the providers of anonymous tissue.

This account of mitochondria is not consonant with current epigenetic research, however, which demonstrates the profound implications of mitochondria with other genetic events in the cell, and their modulation of nuclear DNA (van der Wijst and Rots 2015). Nor is it an adequate account of the extent to which identity is necessarily embodied through collective kinship processes as well as the result of clean filial lines of descent. As the Nuffield report puts it, "Our mitochondrial DNA links us to successive generations of our maternal family rather than to any one individual. The mitochondrial DNA of close relatives such as our mother, brothers and sisters, maternal grandmother, maternal aunts and uncles are likely to be nearly identical, so it would not be possible to identify our mother's mitochondrial DNA from within this group" (Nuffield Council on Bioethics 2012, 19). In other words, the sharing of mitochondria among extended family networks and maternal relations point precisely to the extent that our embodiment, and hence our identity in an affective sense, is a shared quality rather than an effect of possessive individualism.

Moreover, mDNA can only be excluded from considerations of identity if it is defined in such a way that being ill or being healthy are indifferent matters, simply added to or subtracted from a stable self that persists irrespectively. The Nuffield report, in its deliberative sections, acknowledges at some length that this disengagement of identify from health and illness is neither tenable nor defensible.

> The Working Group is . . . sceptical of locating any distinction about the ethical acceptability of interventions on different genomes in notions of identity, because developing a possibly life-limiting disorder (or not) can make such a significant difference to the life of the future person. The Group observed that mitochondrial disorders (or their absence) can affect multiple aspects of identity including self-conception (which may include notions of "genetic identity"), one's bodily identity and social identity, regardless of which genome contains the causative mutations. (Nuffield Council on Bioethics 2012, 57)

Nevertheless, the report advises that mDNA donation should not be acknowledged as reproductive donation, and that the donor should not be recognized through a registry.

So if we consider what is at stake in mDNA therapies in a way that accounts for their affective and communal implications, we could argue that women seek out this treatment precisely because they do not want to inflict their maternal line inheritance of disability and morbidity on their children. They want instead to terminate this aspect of their family inheritance in their own bodies, to stem the flow of mutated mDNA to the next generation. Mitochondrial transplantation enables the donor to divert her own healthy maternal inheritance into the recipient's line of descent, sharing it beyond the boundaries that would normally be created by direct family formation. This channels the generational flows of mitochondria in ways that will create children without these particular disabilities.

What is at stake here is a form of identity, illness, and genetic inheritance that is constituted through the deep time of mitochondrial stability, different from the recombinant novelty of nuclear DNA yet as profoundly implicated in how cellular life informs organism life and human biography. It points to another way to think about the question with which I opened this book—what does it mean to live with a cell lineage? Mitochondrial inheritance brings with it the capacity to live an energetic life, to be viable and equal to the demands of life, and mutations of this inheritance jeopardize and compromise these animal capacities. Such energetic or compromised lives are collective qualities, shared across extensive maternal kinship and up and down the lines of maternal descent, yet they profoundly shape and enable the experience of each person who shares them. They underpin identity not as ex nihilo singularity, but as the iteration of shared biology, as a discrete point within a flow of generational time.

Conclusion

....

Oocytes, more than any other human tissue, conserve the past and create the future. We have seen how they roll up and unfurl different orders of time: evolutionary, ancestral, ontogenic, and biographical. They form the material substrate through which generational time travels, linking each woman's life course back into the deep time of mammalian evolution, family provenance, and matrilineal inheritance, and forward into the lives of children and their descendants. They tick away fertile time for women whose professional aspirations, personal relationships, or economic circumstances cannot be reconciled with the demands of childbearing. While many women do not seek the particular destiny of motherhood, those who do may find that the temporal fragility of their fertility collides with corporate expectations and token gestures to "work-life balance." The unforgiving demands of professional life propel more and more women to seek solutions to this fragility, through egg freezing, IVF, or donation, the technical repertoire of the oocyte economy. As we have seen throughout this book, however, this repertoire cannot entirely compensate for the time-fragile biology of oocytes, and these solutions are often partial, incomplete, or failed.

The structure of feeling I have teased out from the fieldwork informing this study is necessarily shaped by the material constraints and affordances of the oocyte economy, the pragmatics and logistics that limit and shape how oocytes can be procured, exchanged, and accumulated. In this sense it is shaped by the history of reproductive science and of clinical and corporate innovation. It is highly expressive of how IVF and its cognate technologies disaggregate motherhood into an array of maternal agents, whose contribution to any given child is partial and contestable, potentially at least. The oocyte economy *divides and redistributes* raw fertility, renders it storable, portable, transactable, a capacity that can be circulated and leveraged. Yet it cannot be entirely disentangled from the affective dimensions of family obligation and the former biological integrity of the mother-child bond. The logistics remain embedded in the historical specificity of reproductive biopolitics and popular understandings of genetics, gestation, and birth. Hence when the women who contributed to this study speak about their oocytes, they bring all these dimensions into the conversation.

We saw that women who seek fertility treatment quickly find themselves in thrall to the oocyte economy. It is here that they may first realize that their chances of a child depend on the mercurial fertility of their eggs. While many will conceive with their own eggs, more will not. In vitro fertilization and ancillary treatments are the engines of the oocyte economy, creating the deficits and the desires that put the entire economy *in train*. It is here too that women first understand how their identity is bound up with their eggs. Not liberal, individual identity so much as relational identity, a self indebted to a family history and owed to a family future. This realization underpins the determination of fertility patients and women who freeze their eggs, as they struggle to establish their claims in a new generation. It underpins the poignant anxieties expressed by the women whose children were conceived with another woman's eggs.

These sentiments point to a constitutive feature of all tissue economies—they are, necessarily, personified systems. Ex vivo tissues are synecdochal. They stand for the body in which they arise, and they are indelibly marked with the biology and biography of their donor. As Warwick Anderson puts it, they are things with the qualities of persons, and this quality is an intrinsic element of their efficacy (Anderson 2015). We can see this play out in other kinds of tissue donation: the cardiac patient who, near death, is saved by a donor heart and is haunted by gratitude to the unknown benefactor; the fear of some organ recipients that their new kidney or liver is hostile to them, rejecting them and wishing them ill (Waldby 2002); the romantic fantasies some women report about their anonymized sperm donor (Tober 2001). In a more dramatic contemporary example, my extended study of the Visible Human Project (Waldby 2000) explores how the VHP archive is haunted by the identity of the man and woman whose corpses were used to create the images, so that the VHP is simultaneously medical and memorial.

This personification is most acute in relation to reproductive tissues, eggs, sperm, and embryos, precisely because they are tissues that most completely convey the donor, and they are things that may become new persons. They convey not only the singularity of their most proximate donor but that person's ancestral history, and they create new lines of descent. This sense of personification generates the structure of feeling expressed most clearly by the women whose children were donor conceived. They were inundated by a sense that the child was not fully theirs, that they were maternal imposters who fulfilled their obligations to past and future imperfectly. The child, they feared, personified the donor and the donor's lineage, not theirs. They struggled to reconcile their maternal feelings and claims with the imagined claims of the oocyte provider. Not all the women in this group felt this way, however, and we saw some more assertive positions among the interviewees. Molly argued that gestation and nurture trump genetics, while Jo embraced the donor's lineage, seeing it as an antiracist way to celebrate her husband's Asian lineage and Australia's Asian location. Nevertheless, these less defensive positions involved a search for an anonymous donor, and a sense that identified donation would compromise their family's integrity. Jo's sense of affiliation with Southeast Asians, and the converse anxieties among the women who feared the Mediterranean traces that their children might bear, also point toward how oocyte economies play out matters of race, nation, and citizenship. As personified systems, they necessarily bring with themselves not only familial identity but also the social history of white privilege and the processes through which whiteness is reproduced (Cooper and Waldby 2014).

We saw a similar unease and fear of compromised lineage among the women who froze their eggs and the couples interviewed for the HFEA patient consultation about mitochondrial transplant. Personal egg freezing is a way to conserve one's lineage by donating to one's future self. This group of women tried to shape a future when their own eggs could form a basis for uncompromised relations with partner and child. Egg freezing was a welcome alternative to donation. Most felt that they would prefer to remain childless or to adopt if they could not conceive with their own eggs. Adoption was regarded as preferable by some of the interviewees because it was transparent. It would be clear, in most cases, that the child was *not* biologically theirs, so it did not involve an attempt to *conceal* an egg donation, and it could contribute to the well-being of a child already in the world. It offered a degree of ethical redemption, they felt, that was not afforded by donor conception.

Some of the interviewees acknowledged that they may have "left it too late," freezing their eggs in their late thirties. Egg bank staff in the United States and on the UK informed me that younger women, in their mid- or late twenties, were presenting in ever growing numbers to inquire about egg freezing. It seems probable that, for a certain class of young women with sufficient disposable income, this form of self-preservation may become routine. As with other forms of private tissue banking, it may come to be regarded as a prudent form of biological insurance (Waldby 2006; Fannin 2013), a way to hedge one's bets against the uncertainties of career and life course. As high-profile technology companies like Google offer egg freezing as part of a benefits package to their young female hires, we can see how this practice may become normalized and glamourized, simply a sensible form of investment in the future and good professional conduct (see, for example, Bennett 2014).

Women who bank their eggs want to secure the personified aura of the material, to preserve the integrity of the different genetic components and their undivided relationship to themselves. The eggs are invested with the power to keep a desired future intact, one in which the women can elect to have a child whose maternity and generational lineage cannot be in doubt. We can see the converse position among the Australian altruistic donors and the mitochondrial disease focus groups involved in the HFEA consultation (Sheikh 2013). Each of these groups worked to *depersonalize* oocytes, to drain them of all but their mechanical significance. The altruistic donors insisted that their contribution to the child was merely instrumental, a simple biological device whose action did not eclipse the moral claims of the intending mother. This way of framing their contribution could be regarded as an extension of their gift. They give not only the biological material but also a form of words that defers to the feelings of the gestational mother and enhances her priority to the child. Nevertheless, we saw that this preparedness to give was attendant on their vetting of the mother or couple. The donors felt that they should exercise moral agency to ensure that any child resulting from their gift would be loved and cared for. It is evident that they cannot entirely divorce themselves from an investment in the child that their oocytes might become. Their feeling for the potential child is maternal, but at a remove, a second-order ethics of care that seems proportional to what they considered their second-order contribution to the conception. Not all donors will feel this way. The Australian altruistic donors' feelings about their role are informed by the fact that at most Australian clinics, the IVF patient or couple is expected to find the donor. Potential donor and recipient are in a comparatively unmediated relation to each other, and given the scarcity of altruistic donors, any woman prepared to consider such a role will have several possible intending parents from which to choose. In the UK and the United States, clinics and agencies recruit donors. In these circumstances, donors do not play an active part in the matching process, will not be in a position to vet, and cannot exercise the same kind of agency. We saw that even the most professionalized cohorts of egg providers, however, those selected by the Californian clinic, valued the anonymized letters of appreciation and reassurance that their recipients wrote, as a way to feel some personal connection with the outcome.

In the case of mitochondrial donation, the entire logic of the treatment is organized around a mechanical interpretation of oocyte action. Treatment is rhetorically framed to personify nuclear DNA alone, and to depersonalize all other aspects of donated eggs. The mitochondria are simply batteries—neutral, anonymous forms of energy—and they can be added and subtracted without implication for the identity of any child conceived through the technique. This kind of hierarchy gives the mother and father of any child conceived a symmetrical claim. The child can be positioned as the descendant of each parent's lineage, while the donor's lineage can be set aside. It parries the "three-parent embryo" iconography favored by the media, making it seem sensational and alarmist.

Taken together these different ways of construing oocyte action all point toward the difficulty of reconciling the disaggregation of maternal action effected by the oocyte economy. While any given women may contribute to the creation of a child as an intending parent, a reproductive donor, a gestational carrier, or a mitochondrial donor, we can see that immense regulatory and commercial energy and rhetorical inventiveness have been invested in the preservation of a singular mother-child claim and in the protection of normative forms of family formation (Cooper and Waldby 2014). This is evident in the proliferation of contractual forms of donation, where the oocyte provider is an anonymous, external supplier of fertility services to the family proper, and the provider and recipient are quits once the transaction is complete. In the California clinic we saw that this contractual model was enhanced by the organization of the new egg bank, so that young women provided their oocytes to the bank, rather than to a particular commissioning couple. Here we can see that, in contrast to the women who elected to freeze their own eggs, cryopreservation was used to depersonalize, to make provision more like a professional service relation and less like an intimate exchange. It is evident in the careful codification of legitimate and illegitimate maternal claims in the statutes and common law of various jurisdictions, even when the content was widely variable; in Australia the gestational mother has priority, while in California, the intending mother is the legal parent. It is evident too in the vigorous exclusion of mitochondrial donors from recognition in the conception process, in the UK at least. They do *not* create three-parent embryos, we are told, and they are *not* to be registered as reproductive donors.

As we have seen, however, this regulatory and commercial insistence that maternity is a strictly unified, zero-sum status was not necessarily felt as such by the women interviewed for this study. Rather, their anxieties and misgivings point toward an involuntary acknowledgment that the oocyte economy has irrevocably complicated the terrain of maternal action, and that they may always feel that their claim to the child is shared with others, even when the others are unknown and elsewhere. While statutory codification of legal parenthood is necessary for any jurisdiction, strict allocation of maternal rights and obligations around custody and care do not necessarily exclude other kinds of acknowledgment. I would argue that the structure of feeling we can discern here is more adequately represented in a regulatory sense by donor registries. Registries recognize the complications of the oocyte economy, giving forms of recognition to donors that do not infringe on family law matters of custody or access yet provide for the child's interest in knowing their full biological origins. The donor's contribution is a matter of record, and any child conceived may seek information and contact.

The creation of mandatory registries is a regulatory response to the harms that have emerged from twentieth-century adoption practice, the grief articulated by both relinquishing mothers and adopted children at the loss of their possibilities for relationship (Klass, Silverman, and Nickman 1996). Anonymized adoption works on the same zero-sum logic described above, an insistence that the mother-child relation be singular and undivided. This conviction has lessened gradually over the last thirty years, however, as more evidence has emerged of the benefits of adoptive families that acknowledge the birth mother's role and accommodate the child's desire to know their origins. In this same spirit, mandatory registries preserve the possibility of future contact and meet the growing concern regarding genetic lineage, the sense that children should know their family medical history to make good choices about their own health. Registries acknowledge the different kinds of maternal action made possible by the oocyte economy and confer a status on the donor that gives more adequate recognition of this array. At the same time, we have seen that mandatory registries were not welcomed by many of the women interviewed, and some went to considerable lengths to circumvent them, traveling overseas to find egg providers. Registries only operate *within* particular jurisdictions, so their action is national or provincial; they cannot extend to cross-border procurement. The global market for oocytes means that intending mothers may avoid acknowledgment of the egg provider's contribution if they so wish. Nevertheless, their fears that they are not the "true mother" suggests that avoidance does not suffice, and that the egg provider's contribution is more honored in the breach than in the observance.[1]

To return finally to the questions with which I opened this study: What does it mean to live with this cell lineage? What does it mean to participate in the oocyte economy? Clearly, it gives women a wider scope of action for the ordering of their fertility. To paraphrase Hannah Landecker, it changes what it means to be reproductive.[2] Women may use the technologies described in this study to bring their atavistic mammalian biology more happily in line with the demands of credentialing, corporate life, and professional development. They can negotiate to give or sell their own fertility or procure that of another. They can take advantage of the fact that the former unities of place and time that once defined human reproduction have disaggregated across the globe and through time. Yet as we have seen, none of these technical transformations is without social consequence or cost. Egg freezing may simply offer companies another way to deny women adequate maternity leave, while the odds of successful conception with stored eggs may still be poor for women who bank them in their thirties. Egg donation places women into unprecedented, ethically fraught relations with each other and with any resulting child.

The structure of feeling mapped in this study suggests that such relations still lack an ethical language, ways of reasoning about appropriate recognition, including distributive justice, given that most oocyte transactions involve poor providers and well-off recipients. This lack is exacerbated rather than ameliorated by resort to the generic terminology of institutional and regulatory bioethics, wherein the informed consent of the provider is presumed to answer for all questions related to justice (Cooper and Waldby 2014). It is also perpetrated by the DNA centrism evident not only in the interviewees' understandings of gametes and genetics but also in some regulatory discourse, notably that around mitochondrial donation. We saw that in each case the parent-child biological relation is cast as an effect of nuclear DNA, to the exclusion of other kinds of genetic, cytoplasmic, placental, or gestational contributions to the formation of the neonate. This way of framing parent-child biology may give comfort to mothers wishing to conceive with a mitochondrial donor, yet it necessarily excludes all aspects of women's reproductive capacity other than those that correspond to the action of sperm. If women feel that their donor-conceived child is not "theirs," this arises in part because the nuclear genetic material is privileged over other aspects of gamete action, including, for example, how oocyte biology initiates the placental and uterine conditions of gestation. While a fertile oocyte is needed to set the initial conditions, the recipient's reproductive biology is fully engaged in bringing the conception to full development and birth. A privileging of nuclear DNA is detrimental to women who participate in the oocyte economy. It is detrimental also to a feminist interest in opening out the terms of reproductive science and medicine to a more generous acknowledgment of the complexity of women's biology and the multiple affiliations it may sustain. This study, I hope, is a form of redress, and a means of acknowledgment, a contribution to a more adequate way for us to understand the relations between biological and historical life and how reproductive capacity links one to the other.

Appendix

....

Nonprofessional Interview Participants

(Pseudonyms)

Australian Former IVF Patients

PHILIPPA was in a de facto relationship and had one child. She was in her late forties, had a postgraduate degree, and was a media producer.

CAROLINE was married with no children and was in her early thirties. She had a certificate-level qualification and worked in sales.

EVA was married with one child and was in her early thirties. She had a postgraduate degree and was a public school teacher.

ISABEL was married with one child and was in her late thirties. She had an advanced diploma and worked in marketing.

REBECCA was married with two children and was in her early to mid-thirties. She had a bachelor's degree and was a nurse.

TILLY was married with two children and was in her mid- to late thirties. She had a certificate-level qualification and was a stay-at-home mother.

FRANCESCA was married with one child and was in her late twenties. She had an advanced diploma and was a travel consultant.

JOANNA was married with no children and was in her late twenties. She had completed secondary education and was an insurance professional.

MIRA was married with one child and was in her early thirties. She had completed secondary education and was a home worker.

NADIA was married with one child and was in her late twenties. She had an advanced diploma and was a student.

SARAH was married with one child and was in her late thirties. She had a bachelor's degree and was an accountant.

DOMINIQUE was in a de facto relationship and had no children. She was in her mid-thirties, had a bachelor's degree, and was a chef.

BRIDGET was married with one child and pregnant. She was in her early forties, had completed secondary education, and was a shop assistant.

JERRIE was married with no children and was in her early to mid-thirties. She had a certificate-level qualification and was on a disability pension.

ANNETTE was married with two children and pregnant. She was in her mid- to late thirties, had a graduate diploma, and was a stay-at-home mother.

ROSALIND was married with no children and was in her early to mid-forties. She had a postgraduate degree and was a financial assistant.

DENISE was married with no children and was in her early to mid-thirties. She had a certificate-level qualification and was an office manager.

MANDY was married with no children and in her mid-thirties. She was a nurse and had a bachelor's degree.

MELISSA was married with two children and pregnant. She was in her mid- to late thirties. She had a postgraduate degree and was a social worker.

LISA was married with no children and was in her early to mid-forties. She had an advanced diploma and was a nurse.

Australian Altruistic Donors

AGNES was in a de facto relationship and had no children. She was in her late twenties. She had a bachelor's degree and was an early childhood teacher.

JANE was in a relationship and had no children. She was in her early to mid-thirties. She had completed secondary education and was working in maintenance.

MEG was married with one child and pregnant. She was in her early thirties. She had a postgraduate degree and was a teacher.

SERENA was married with two children and was in her mid-thirties. She had a graduate diploma and was a student.

CHRISTINE was engaged and had no children. She was in her early thirties. She had a certificate-level qualification and was a homecare nurse.

British Women Who Traveled Overseas to Seek Oocyte Providers

BELINDA was married with one child and was between forty-six and fifty years old. She had an advanced diploma and was a home worker.

LEILA was married with two children and was between forty-one and forty-five years old. She had completed secondary education and was an office manager.

OLIVIA was single with no children and was between forty-six and fifty years old. She had a bachelor's degree and worked as a media professional.

RACHEL was married with one child and was between forty-one and forty-five years old. She had completed secondary education and was a bank director.

Australian Women Who Traveled Overseas to Seek Oocyte Providers

KATE was married with one child and was between forty-one and forty-five years old. She had a postgraduate degree and was a lawyer.

ERINNA was married with four children and was between forty-one and forty-five years old. She had a postgraduate degree and was a policy advisor.

MOLLY was single with three children and was between fifty-one and fifty-five years old. She had a postgraduate degree and was an economist.

MIRANDA was in a de facto relationship and had no children but was pregnant. She was between thirty-six and forty years old, had a bachelor's degree, and worked in social media.

JO was married with no children and was between forty-one and forty-five years old. She had a postgraduate degree and was an academic.

British Women Who Froze Their Oocytes

JENNIFER was in a de facto relationship and was in her early forties. She had a bachelor's degree and was a company director.

LOUISE was single and in her late thirties. She had a bachelor's degree and was a PA in the finance sector.

AVA was single with one child and was in her early forties. She had a postgraduate degree and was a media producer.

MICHELLE was in a de facto relationship and was in her late twenties. She had a bachelor's degree and was a police officer.

PHOEBE was in a same-sex relationship and was in her late thirties. She had a bachelor's degree and was an engineer.

VERONICA was single and in her late thirties. She had a postgraduate degree and was a charity organizational professional.

ANITA was single and was in her early forties. She had a postgraduate degree and was a director of her own business.

NAOMI was in a de facto relationship and was in her late thirties. She had a bachelor's degree and worked for a recruitment consultancy.

FAITH was single and was in her mid- to late thirties. She had a postgraduate degree and was a lawyer.

URSULA was in a de facto relationship and was in her early to mid-forties. She had a bachelor's degree and was a business owner.

ALISON was in a new de facto relationship and was in her early forties. She had a bachelor's degree and was an IT project manager.

ELEANOR was in a de facto relationship, pregnant, and in her early thirties. She had a postgraduate degree and was a business relationship manager.

FLORENCE was single and was in her mid- to late thirties. She had a bachelor's degree and was a TV producer.

THEA was single and in her mid-thirties. She had a bachelor's degree and was a journalist.

MEREDITH was single and in her early thirties. She had a postgraduate degree and was an occupational therapist.

Australian Young Women's Focus Group Participants

ROSEANNE was in her mid-twenties. She had a bachelor's degree and was studying nursing.

CARA was in her late twenties. She had a postgraduate degree and was a postdoctoral medical research scientist.

DELIA was in her late twenties. She had a bachelor's degree and was working as a research assistant in nursing.

DONNA was in her early twenties. She was an undergraduate student and a retail assistant.

ERICA was in her mid-twenties. She had a bachelor's degree and was a dietician.

FRANCINE was in her mid-twenties. She was an undergraduate student and majoring in law.

EVELINE was in her early twenties. She was an undergraduate student studying psychology.

MONA was in her early twenties. She was an undergraduate student studying psychology.

VANESSA was in her mid-twenties. She had a bachelor's degree and was studying medicine.

CELESTE was in her mid-twenties. She was an undergraduate student in psychology and arts.

VIOLET was in her early twenties. She was an undergraduate student in media and communication.

GISELLE was in her early twenties. She had completed secondary education and was studying psychology.

ALBERTINE was in her mid-twenties. She had a bachelor's degree majoring in ancient history.

MARTHA was in her mid- to late twenties. She was a doctoral student in social science.

Notes

....

Introduction

1   In Australia, for example, between 2007 and 2008, 55 percent of births were to women aged thirty to thirty-nine, with a significant proportion to women over thirty-five (Kuleshova 2009). In Britain the number of live births to mothers aged forty or over has nearly tripled between 1990 and 2010 (Mullen 2011).

2   Catherine Waldby, Ian Kerridge, and Loane Skene, CIS, 2008–2011, "Human oöcytes for stem cell research: Donation and regulation in Australia," ARC Linkage Project—LP0882054.

3   Catherine Waldby, CI, 2011–2015, "The oöcyte economy: The hanging meanings of human eggs in fertility, assisted reproduction and stem cell research," ARC Future Fellowship—FT100100176.

4   Notably, all but one participant was heterosexual. I have drawn on secondary literature to flesh out points of comparison with the dynamics of same-sex relationships.

5 Hwang Woo Suk and his research team published two fraudulent papers in *Science* (in 2004 and 2005) falsely claiming to have created the world's first human SCNT cell lines in their South Korean laboratories. When the fraud was identified, in 2005, investigators also discovered that the team had procured more than two thousand oocytes from paid providers and some from the laboratory researchers. I discuss this case in more detail in chapter 7.

6 Margaret Boulos, Kim McLeod, and Brydan Leanne also conducted some interviews. In addition, Margaret Boulos conducted the focus groups for young nonpatient women.

7 Lemke's quote from Foucault can be found in volume 2 of *The History of Sexuality* (Foucault 1990, 4).

8 Lost in English but retained in modern French. Thanks to Michelle Jamison for bringing this point to my attention.

9 See, for example, Henderson (2014).

One. Temporal Oocytes

1 In human beings, a typical sperm is 5 to 7 μm long, while the diameter of the ovum is twenty times that size.

2 "Cloning" is a term that refers to many forms of in vivo and in vitro cell division in biology, so I use SCNT throughout as a far more specific descriptor for the process that produced Dolly.

Two. Twentieth-Century Oocytes

1 "From 50.7 conceptions resulting in live births per 1,000 unmarried women aged 15 to 44 in 1971, the overall total rate of nonmarital conception plummeted to 29.7 in 1976" (Carmichael 1996, 302).

2 Single, never-married mother households increased from 1.2 percent of all families in the UK in 1970 to 8 percent in 1994 (Kiernan, Land, and Lewis 1998).

3 "Abandoned tissue" is the term used historically to characterize tissue excised during surgical procedures and made available to researchers without the need for formal consent. For a discussion of this category, see Waldby and Mitchell (2006).

4 Haldane's speculative work, *Daedalus, or, Science and the Future*, presented at Cambridge in 1923, proposed the virtues of "ectogenesis," human reproduction in the laboratory rather than in vivo, and was an influence on Aldous Huxley's *Brave New World* (Clarke 1998).

Three. Precious Oocytes

1 "A woman's age affects her fertility," Your Fertility, accessed January 2, 2015, http://yourfertility.org.au/for-women/age.
2 Intracytoplasmic sperm injection involves the injection of a single sperm directly into a mature egg. It is used in cases of male infertility.
3 Australia does not have a compulsory disposal date for cryopreserved embryos.
4 Although courts may order transfer of parentage in cases of surrogacy. See the New South Wales Surrogacy Act 2010, for example.

Four. Global Oocytes

1 See the Commonwealth's *Family Law Act 1975. Different states in Australia* have enacted additional legislation to facilitate transfer of maternal parentage from birth mother to intending parent in cases of lawful (i.e., noncommercial) surrogacy, such as the *Surrogacy Act 2010* (NSW). In the UK, the birth mother is automatically recognized as the legal mother under common law and embedded in the Human Fertilisation and Embryology (HFE) Act 2008. For California law, see Surrogacy Agreements AB1217 (2013).
2 In Victoria, donor registries are mandated by the Assisted Reproductive Treatment Act 2008 and the Assisted Reproductive Treatment Regulations 2009. In New South Wales, they fall under the Assisted Reproductive Technology Act 2007 and Assisted Reproductive Technology Regulation 2009. In the UK the HFEA administers mandatory donor registries under the Human Fertilisation and Embryology Act 1990.
3 See chapter 7 for details of the Hwang scandal.
4 See the Act on the Protection of Embryos (Embryonenschutzgesetz [ESchG]) of December 13, 1990, *Bundesgesetzblatt*, part I, 1990, pp. 2746–2748, amended by article 1 of the act of November 21, 2011 (*Bundesgesetzblatt*, part I, 2011, p. 2228), which forbids the creation of supernumerary embryos.
5 See "Access to donor information around the world," Health Law Central, accessed November 10, 2017, http://www.healthlawcentral.com/donorconception/international-laws-access-donor-information.
6 The Al Aqsa Intifada was the second Intifada, or Palestinian uprising against Israel, 2000 to 2005.

Five. Cold-Chain Oocytes

1 See, for example, Johnston and Zoll (2014) and Brow (2015).
2 U.S. clinics use standardized instruments like the Minnesota Multiphasic Personality Inventory, which screens for personality and mental health disorders.

3   See the Cryoport home page, accessed November 28, 2016, http://www.cryoport
    .com.

4   By 2013, it was estimated that these clinics between them held approximately
    3,130 oocytes from 294 donors. Since the first bank was founded in 2004, these
    facilities have carried out about 1,500 transfer cycles using frozen oocytes,
    resulting in 602 pregnancies by 2012.

5   In Australia, the Prohibition of Human Cloning for Reproduction Act 2002
    makes it an offense to "intentionally give, receive or offer to give or receive valu-
    able consideration for the supply of a human egg, human sperm or a human
    embryo. . . . Valuable consideration, in relation to the supply of a human egg,
    human sperm or a human embryo by a person, includes any inducement,
    discount or priority in the provision of a service to the person." In the UK, the
    Human Fertilisation and Embryology (HFE) Act 1990, states that "no money
    or other benefit shall be given or received in respect of any supply of gametes,
    embryos or human admixed embryos." The act has been subsequently modi-
    fied by the Gamete and Embryo Donation Ref: 0001 to include compensation
    of up to £750 for oocyte donors. The UK is also bound by several EU instru-
    ments that forbid the exchange of human tissues for money, including the Tis-
    sues and Cells Directive (Directive 2004/23/EC) and the Oviedo Convention.

6   See the VARTA guidelines on importation of gametes: Victorian Assisted Repro-
    ductive Treatment Authority (2013).

Six. Private Oocytes

1   "Advanced clinic search," Human Fertilisation and Embryology Authority,
    accessed August 1, 2018, http://guide.hfea.gov.uk/guide/.

Seven. Innovation Oocytes

1   The Thylacine Museum, 5th ed., accessed October 12, 2016, http://www.natural
    worlds.org/thylacine.

2   "Newcastle awarded world's first mitochondrial licence," press release, March 16,
    2017, accessed March 2, 2018, http://www.ncl.ac.uk/press/news/2017/03/mito
    chondrialicence.

3   See, for example, Kristol and Cohen (2002), a collection of U.S. conservative
    commentary on the dystopian effects of human cloning.

4   At time of writing, the list of countries that legislate to permit therapeutic clon-
    ing includes some states in the United States, the UK, Canada, Mexico, Co-
    lumbia, Belgium, Finland, Spain, Sweden, China, Taiwan, Japan, Singapore,
    South Korea, Thailand, Australia, New Zealand, Israel, Iran, and Turkey. See
    Slabbert and Pepper (2015).

5   Note that this was not an entirely consensus position among the feminists involved in the debate. See Charis Thompson's (2007) intervention "Why we should, in fact, pay for egg donation."

6   See, for example, MITOMAP: *A Human Mitochondrial Genome Database*, accessed January 27, 2016, http://www.mitomap.org/MITOMAP.

7   "Human fertilisation and embryology act 2008," legislation.gov.uk, The National Archives, accessed February 3, 2016, http://www.legislation.gov.uk/ukpga /2008/22/enacted.

8   "On human gene editing: International summit statement," The National Academies of Sciences, Engineering, Medicine, December 3, 2015, accessed October 26, 2018, http://www8.nationalacademies.org/onpinews/newsitem .aspx?RecordID=12032015a.

9   See, for example, Boyle (2015).

10 "Mitochondrial donation," The Lily Foundation, accessed February 26, 2018, https://www.thelilyfoundation.org.uk/get-informed/mitochondrial-donation.

11 "Healing broken batteries: The Wellcome Trust Centre for Mitochondrial Research," film by Barry J. Gibb, Youtube.com, September 15, 2012, accessed October 26, 2018, https://www.youtube.com/watch?v=Sr7Jnr9qn44.

Conclusion

1   Research with donor-conceived adults who discover their status only when they are adolescent or adult suggests that late disclosure does have a detrimental effect on the parent-child bond. Donor-conceived adults report being angrier with their mothers for late disclosure than with their fathers, while donor-conceived children informed in childhood report a more positive regard for the situation (Jadva, Freeman, and Kramer 2009).

2   "Biotechnology changes what it is to be biological" (Landecker 2005, n.p.).

References

....

Alichniewicz, A., and M. Michałowska. 2015. "Challenges to ART market: A Polish case." *Medicine, Health Care, and Philosophy* 18: 141–146.

Almeling, R. 2011. *Sex Cells: The Medical Market in Eggs and Sperm*. Berkeley: University of California Press.

Almeling, R., and I. L. Willey. 2017. "Same medicine, different reasons: Comparing women's bodily experiences of producing eggs for pregnancy or for profit." *Social Science and Medicine* 188: 21–29.

Amato, P., M. Tachibana, M. Sparman, and S. Mitalipov. 2014. "Three-parent in vitro fertilization: Gene replacement for the prevention of inherited mitochondrial diseases." *Fertility and Sterility* 101 (1): 31–35.

American Society for Reproductive Medicine. 2013. "Mature oocyte cryopreservation: A guideline." *Fertility and Sterility* 99 (1): 37–43.

Andersen, A. N., V. Goossens, S. Bhattacharya, A. P. Ferraretti, M. S. Kupka, J. de Mouzon, and K. G. Nygren. 2009. "Assisted reproductive technology and intrauterine inseminations in Europe, 2005: Results generated from European registers by ESHRE." *Human Reproduction* 24 (6): 1267–1287.

Anderson, W. 2005. *The Cultivation of Whiteness: Science, Health and Racial Destiny in Australia*. Carlton, Vic.: Melbourne University Press.

Anderson, W. 2008. *The Collectors of Lost Souls: Turning Kuru Scientists into Whitemen*. Baltimore, MD: Johns Hopkins University Press.

Anderson, W. 2015. "The frozen archive, or defrosting Derrida." *Journal of Cultural Economy* 8 (3): 379–387.

Australia in the Asian Century Task Force. 2012. *Australia in the Asian century: White Paper*. Canberra: Commonwealth of Australia.

Bavister, B. D. 2002. "Early history of in vitro fertilization." *Reproduction* 124: 181–196.

Becker, G. S. 1993. *Human Capital: A Theoretical and Empirical Analysis with Special Reference to Education*. Chicago: University of Chicago Press.

Beckles, H. 1989. *Natural Rebels: A Social History of Enslaved Black Woman in Barbados*. London: Zed Books.

Benjamin, R. 2013. *People's Science Bodies and Rights on the Stem Cell Frontier*. Palo Alto, CA: Stanford University Press.

Benjamin, W. (1935) 1968. "The work of art in the age of mechanical reproduction." In *Illuminations*, edited by Hannah Arendt, 217–251. New York: Harcourt.

Bennett, J. 2014. "Company-paid egg freezing will be the great equalizer." *Time*, October 15, 2014. http://time.com/3509930/company-paid-egg-freezing-will -be-the-great-equalizer/.

Bergmann, S. 2011a. "Fertility tourism: Circumventive routes that enable access to reproductive technologies and substances." *Signs* 36 (2): 280–289.

Bergmann, S. 2011b. "Reproductive agency and projects: Germans searching for egg donation in Spain and the Czech Republic." *Reproductive BioMedicine Online* 23 (5): 600–608.

Bergmann, S. 2012. "Resemblance that matters. On transnational anonymized egg donation in two European IVF clinics." In *Reproductive Technologies as Global Form: Ethnographies of Knowledge, Practices, and Transnational Encounters*, edited by Michi Knecht, Maren Klotz, and Stefan Beck, 331–355. Frankfurt: Campus Verlag.

Bergson, H., and A. Mitchell. 1911. *Creative Evolution*. New York: Holt.

Berry, E. R. 2008. "The zombie commodity: Hair and the politics of its globalization." *Postcolonial Studies* 11 (1): 63–84.

Biggers, J. D. 1991. "Walter Heape, FRS, a pioneer in reproductive biology: Centenary of his embryo transfer experiments." *Journal of Reproduction and Fertility* 93: 172–186.

Blyth, E. 2002. "Subsidized IVF: The development of 'egg sharing' in the UK." *Human Reproduction* 17 (12): 3254–3259.

Bonner, J. F. 1965. *The Molecular Biology of Development*. New York: Oxford University Press.

Boston Women's Health Book Collective. 1973. *Our Bodies, Ourselves*. New York: Simon and Schuster.

Boulos, M. 2014. "Scientific utilisations of reproductive tissues: 'Good eggs,' women and altruism." PhD diss., University of Sydney.

Boulos, M., I. Kerridge, and C. Waldby. 2014. "Reciprocity in the donation of reproductive oöcytes." In *Reframing Reproduction: Conceiving Gendered Experience in Late Modernity*, edited by M. Nash, 203–220. London: Palgrave Macmillan.

Boyle, Darren. 2015. "UK becomes first country in the world to legalise three-parent babies after Lords approves controversial IVF technique." *Daily Mail*, February 25, 2015. http://www.dailymail.co.uk/news/article-2967544/UK-country-world-legalise-three-parent-babies-Lords-approves-controversial-IVF-technique.html.

Braun, K., and S. Schultz. 2012. "Oöcytes for research: Inspecting the commercialization continuum." *New Genetics and Society* 31 (2): 135–157.

Brow, Jason. 2015. "Khloe Kardashian freezing her eggs? She admits Kim has talked with her about it." *Hollywood Life*, November 3, 2015. http://hollywoodlife.com/2015/11/03/khloe-kardashian-freezing-eggs-kim-pregnancy-kids/.

Brown, N., and A. Kraft. 2006. "Blood ties: Banking the stem cell promise." *Technology Analysis and Strategic Management* 18 (3/4): 313–327.

Bühler, N. 2015. "Imagining the future of motherhood: The medically assisted extension of fertility and the production of genealogical continuity." *Sociologus* 65 (1): 79–100.

Byrd, L. M., M. Sidebotham, and B. Lieberman. 2002. "Egg donation—the donor's view: An aid to future recruitment." *Human Fertility* 5 (4): 175–182.

Canguilhem, G. 2008. *Knowledge of Life*. Edited by P. Marrati, and T. Meyers. New York: Fordham University Press.

Carmichael, G. A. 1996. "From floating brothels to suburban semirespectability: Two centuries of nonmarital pregnancy in Australia." *Journal of Family History* 21 (3): 281–315.

Carroll, K. 2013. "Infertile? The emotional labour of sensitive and feminist research methodologies." *Qualitative Research* 13 (5): 546–561.

Carroll, K., and C. Waldby. 2012. "Informed consent and fresh egg donation for stem cell research." *Journal of Bioethical Inquiry* 9 (1): 29–39.

Castiaux, E. 2011. "Introduction to cold chain management—part II." *Journal of GXP Compliance* 15 (1): 49–53.

Centers for Disease Control and Prevention. 2017. "2015 Assisted reproductive technology fertility clinic success rates report." Atlanta, GA: U.S. Department of Health and Human Services.

Chambers, G. M., V. P. Hoang, and P. J. Illingworth. 2013. "Socioeconomic disparities in access to ART treatment and the differential impact of a policy that increased consumer costs." *Human Reproduction* 28 (11): 3111–3117.

Chang, M. C. 1959. "Fertilization of rabbit ova in vitro." *Nature* 184 (4684): 466–467.

Chen, C. 1986. "Pregnancy after human oocyte cryopreservation." *Lancet* 1: 884–886.

Chian, R.-C., Y. Wang, and Y.-R. Li. 2014. "Oocyte vitrification: Advances, progress and future goals." *Journal of Assisted Reproduction and Genetics* 31 (4): 411–420.

Chisholm, R. 2012. "Information rights and donor conception: Lessons from adoption?" *Journal of Law and Medicine* 19: 722–741.

Chrulew, M. 2017. "Freezing the ark: The cryopolitics of endangered species preservation." In *Cryopolitics: Frozen Life in a Melting World*, edited by J. Radin and E. Kowal, 283–306. Cambridge, MA: MIT Press.

Clarke, A. 1998. *Disciplining Reproduction: Modernity, American Life Sciences, and the Problems of Sex*. Berkeley: University of California Press.

Clarke, A. E. 2007. "Reflections on the reproductive sciences in agriculture in the UK and U.S., ca. 1900–2000+." *Studies in History and Philosophy of Science Part C: Studies in History and Philosophy of Biological and Biomedical Sciences* 38 (2): 316–339.

Cobo, A., M. Meseguer, J. Remohi, and A. Pellicer. 2010. "Use of cryo-banked oocytes in an ovum donation programme: A prospective, randomized, controlled, clinical trial." *Human Reproduction* 25 (9): 2239–2246.

Cohen, J., M. Alikani, and S. Franklin. 2015. "The Oldham Notebooks: A look back at one of the most remarkable scientific collaborations of the twentieth century." *Reproductive Biomedicine and Society Online* 1 (1): 1–2.

Cohen, J., A. Trounson, K. Dawson, H. Jones, J. Hazekamp, K. Nygren, and L. Hamberger. 2005. "The early days of IVF outside the UK." *Human Reproduction Update* 11 (5): 439–460.

Colebrook, C. 2009. "Stratigraphic time, women's time." *Australian Feminist Studies* 24 (59): 11–16.

Commonwealth of Australia. 2008. *Families in Australia: 2008*. Canberra: Department of the Prime Minister and Cabinet.

Connor, S. 2015. "Scientist who pioneered 'three-parent' IVF embryo technique now wants to offer it to older women trying for a baby." *Independent Online*, February 8, 2015.

Cooper, E. L. 1976. "Evolution of blood cells." *Annals of Immunology* 127 (6): 817–825.

Cooper, M., and C. Waldby. 2014. *Clinical Labor: Tissue Donors and Research Subjects in the Global Bioeconomy*. Durham, NC: Duke University Press.

Cooper, T. G., E. Noonan, S. von Eckardstein, J. Auger, H. W. G. Baker, H. M. Behre, T. B. Haugen, T. Kruger, C. Wang, M. T. Mbizvo, and K. M. Vogelsong. 2010. "World Health Organization reference values for human semen characteristics." *Human Reproduction Update* 16 (3): 231–245.

Council of Europe. 1997. *Convention for the Protection of Human Rights and Dignity of the Human Being with Regard to the Application of Biology and Medicine.* Convention on Human Rights and Biomedicine, Oviedo, Spain, April 4, 1997. European Treaty Series 164. Strasbourg: Council of Europe.

Cox, P. 2011. "Introduction: The evolutionary mystery of gamete dimorphism." In *The Evolution of Anisogamy: A Fundamental Phenomenon Underlying Sexual Selection,* edited by T. Togashi and P. Cox, 1–16. Cambridge: Cambridge University Press.

Cree, L., and P. Loi. 2015. "Mitochondrial replacement: From basic research to assisted reproductive technology portfolio tool—technicalities and possible risks." *Molecular Human Reproduction* 21 (1): 3–10.

Culley, L., N. Hudson, F. Rapport, E. Blyth, W. Norton, and A. A. Pacey. 2011. "Crossing borders for fertility treatment: Motivations, destinations and outcomes of UK fertility travellers." *Human Reproduction* 26 (9): 2373–2381.

Davy, D. 2014. "Understanding the complexities of responding to child sex trafficking in Thailand and Cambodia." *International Journal of Sociology and Social Policy* 34 (11/12): 793–816.

De Kretzer, D., P. Dennis, B. Hudson, J. Leeton, A. Lopata, K. Outch, J. Talbot, and C. Wood. 1973. "Transfer of a human zygote." *Lancet* 302 (7831): 728–729.

Dickenson, D. 2004. "The threatened trade in human ova." *Nature Reviews Genetics* 5:167–168.

Dickenson, D., and I. A. Idiakez. 2008. "Ova donation for stem cell research: An international perspective." *International Journal of Feminist Approaches to Bioethics* 1 (2): 125–143.

Dodds, S. 2003. "Women, commodification, and embryonic stem-cell research." In *Biomedical Ethics Reviews: Stem Cell Research,* edited by J. Humber and R. F. Almeder, 149–174. Totowa, NJ: Humana Press.

Downie, J., and F. Baylis. 2013. "Transnational trade in human eggs: Law, policy, and (in)action in Canada." *Journal of Law, Medicine and Ethics* 41 (1): 224–239.

Dupré, J. 2012. *Processes of Life: Essays in the Philosophy of Biology.* Oxford: Oxford University Press.

Duranthon, V., and J.-P. Renard. 2003. "Storage and functional recovery of molecules in oocytes." *Biology and Pathology of the Oocyte: Role in Fertility and Reproductive Medicine,* edited by A. Trounson and R. Godsen, 81–112. Cambridge: Cambridge University Press.

Dyer, S., G. M. Chambers, J. de Mouzon, K. G. Nygren, F. Zegers-Hochschild, R. Mansour, O. Ishihara, M. Banker, and G. D. Adamson. 2016. "International Committee for Monitoring Assisted Reproductive Technologies world report: Assisted reproductive technology 2008, 2009 and 2010." *Human Reproduction* 31 (7): 1588–1609.

Edwards, R. G. 1965. "Maturation in vitro of human ovarian oocytes." *Lancet* 286 (7419): 926–929.

Edwards, R. G., B. D. Bavister, and P. C. Steptoe. 1969. "Early stages of fertilization in vitro of human oocytes matured in vitro." *Nature* 221 (5181): 632–635.

Edwards, R. G., and P. C. Steptoe. 1980. *A Matter of Life: The Story of a Medical Breakthrough*. London: Hutchinson.

Elder, K., and M. H. Johnson. 2015a. "The Oldham Notebooks: An analysis of the development of IVF 1969–1978, II: The treatment cycles and their outcomes." *Reproductive Biomedicine and Society Online* 1 (1): 9–18.

Elder, K., and M. H. Johnson. 2015b. "The Oldham Notebooks: An analysis of the development of IVF 1969–1978, IV: Ethical aspects." *Reproductive Biomedicine and Society Online* 1 (1): 34–35.

Ellen, B. 2014. "All this fertility paranoia does women no good." *Guardian* (Manchester), October 5, 2014.

ESHRE Task Force on Ethics and Law, W. Dondorp, G. de Wert, G. Pennings, F. Shenfield, P. Devroey, B. Tarlatzis, P. Barri, and K. Diedrich. 2012. "Oocyte cryopreservation for age-related fertility loss." *Human Reproduction* 27 (5): 1231–1237.

Ethics Committee of the American Society for Reproductive Medicine. 2007. "Financial compensation of oocyte donors." *Fertility and Sterility* 88 (2): 305–309.

Faddy, M., and R. Godsen. 2003. "Modelling the dynamics of ovarian follicle utilization throughout life." In *Biology and Pathology of the Oocyte: Role in Fertility and Reproductive Medicine*, edited by A. Trounson and R. Godsen, 44–52. Cambridge: Cambridge University Press.

Faddy, M. J., R. G. Gosden, A. Gougeon, S. J. Richardson, and J. F. Nelson. 1992. "Accelerated disappearance of ovarian follicles in mid-life: Implications for forecasting menopause." *Human Reproduction* 7 (10): 1342–1346.

Fannin, M. 2013. "The hoarding economy of endometrial stem cell storage." *Body and Society* 19 (4): 32–60.

Fidler, A., and J. Bernstein. 1999. "Infertility: From a personal to a public health problem." *Public Health Reports* 114 (6): 494–511.

Foohey, P. 2010. "Paying women for their eggs for use in stem cell research." *Pace Law Review* 30 (3): 900–926.

Foucault, M. 1978. *The History of Sexuality*. Vol. 1. New York: Vintage Books.

Foucault, M. 1990. *The History of Sexuality.* Vol. 2, *The Use of Pleasure.* New York: Vintage.

France, L. 2006. "Passport, tickets, sun cream, sperm." *Observer* (London), January 15, 2006.

Franklin, S. 2007. *Dolly Mixtures: The Remaking of Genealogy.* Durham, NC: Duke University Press.

Franklin, S. 2013. *Biological Relatives: IVF, Stem Cells, and the Future of Kinship.* Durham, NC: Duke University Press.

Friese, C. 2013. *Cloning Wild Life Zoos, Captivity, and the Future of Endangered Animals.* New York: New York University Press.

Gaudillière, J.-P. 2007. "The farm and the clinic: An inquiry into the making of our biotechnological modernity." *Studies in History and Philosophy of Science Part C: Studies in History and Philosophy of Biological and Biomedical Sciences* 38 (2): 521–529.

Gottlieb, K. 1998. "Human biological samples and the law of property: The trust as a model for biological repositories." In *Stored Tissue Samples: Ethical, Legal and Public Policy Implications,* edited by R. Weir, 182–197. Iowa City: University of Iowa Press.

Gottweis, H., B. Salter, and C. Waldby. 2009. *The Global Politics of Human Embryonic Stem Cell Science: Regenerative Medicine in Transition.* Basingstoke: Palgrave.

Grosz, E. A. 2011. *Becoming Undone: Darwinian Reflections on Life, Politics, and Art.* Durham, NC: Duke University Press.

Gunby, J., F. Bissonnette, C. Librach, and L. Cowan. 2010. "Assisted reproductive technologies (ART) in Canada: 2006 results from the Canadian ART Register." *Fertility and Sterility* 93 (7): 2189–2201.

Gutstein, D. E., F. Y. Liu, M. B. Meyers, A. Choo, and G. I. Fishman. 2003. "The organization of adherens junctions and desmosomes at the cardiac intercalated disc is independent of gap junctions." *Journal of Cell Science* 116: 875–885.

Haimes, E., and K. Taylor. 2009. "Fresh embryo donation for human embryonic stem cell (hESC) research: The experiences and values of IVF couples asked to be embryo donors." *Human Reproduction* 24 (9): 2142–2150.

Haimes, E., and K. Taylor. 2015. "Rendered invisible? The absent presence of egg providers in UK debates on the acceptability of research and therapy for mitochondrial disease." *Monash Bioethics Review* 33 (4): 1–19.

Hamzelou, J. 2016. "World's first baby born with new '3 parent' technique." *New Scientist,* October 1, 2016.

Hartman, C. W., and S. Carnochan. 2002. *City for Sale: The Transformation of San Francisco.* Berkeley: University of California Press.

Harvey, P. A., and L. A. Leinwand. 2011. "Cellular mechanisms of cardiomyopa-thy." *Journal of Cell Biology* 194 (3): 355–365.

Hass, N. 2011. "Time to chill? Egg-freezing technology offers women a chance to extend their fertility. *Vogue*, April 28, 2011. https://www.vogue.com /article/time-to-chill-egg-freezing-technology-offers-a-chance-to-extend -fertility.

Healey, J. 2014 "Babies in your 30s? Don't worry, your great-grandma did it too." *The Conversation*, December 19, 2014. http://theconversation.com/babies-in -your-30s-dont-worry-your-great-grandma-did-it-too-34273.

Healy, K. J. 2006. *Last Best Gifts: Altruism and the Market for Human Blood and Organs.* Chicago: University of Chicago Press.

Heidegger, M. 1977. *The Question Concerning Technology, and Other Essays.* New York: Harper and Row.

Hellebrekers, D. M., R. Wolfe, A. T. Hendrickx, I. F. de Coo, C. E. de Die, J. P. Geraedts, P. F. Chinnery, and H. J. Smeets. 2012. "PGD and heteroplasmic mitochondrial DNA point mutations: A systematic review estimating the chance of healthy offspring." *Human Reproduction Update* 18 (4): 341–349.

Henderson, J. M. 2014. "Why we should be alarmed that Apple and Facebook are paying for employee egg freezing." *Forbes Online*, October 15, 2014. https:// www.forbes.com/sites/jmaureenhenderson/2014/10/15/dont-work-for-or -trust-a-company-that-pays-you-to-freeze-your-eggs/#4129622d1c9a.

Herbert, D., J. Lucke, and A. Dobson. 2009. "Infertility, medical advice and treatment with fertility hormones and/or in vitro fertilisation: A population perspective from the Australian Longitudinal Study on Women's Health." *Australian and New Zealand Journal of Public Health* 33 (4): 358–364.

Holliday, R., D. Bell, O. Cheung, M. Jones, and E. Probyn. 2015. "Brief encoun-ters: Assembling cosmetic surgery tourism." *Social Science and Medicine* 124: 298–304.

Hopwood, N. 2000. "Producing development: The anatomy of human embryos and the norms of Wilhelm His." *Bulletin of the History of Medicine* 74 (1): 29–79.

Human Fertilisation and Embryology Authority. 1998. *Cloning Issues in Reproduction, Science and Medicine.* London: Human Genetics Advisory Commission.

Human Fertilisation and Embryology Authority. 2013. *Mitochondria Replace-ment Consultation: Advice to Government.* London: Human Fertilisation and Embryology Authority.

Human Fertilisation and Embryology Authority. 2015a. *Code of Practice.* 8th ed. London: Human Fertilisation and Embryology Authority.

Human Fertilisation and Embryology Authority. 2015b. *Fertility Treatment in 2013: Trends and Figures.* London: Human Fertilisation and Embryology Authority.

Human Fertilisation and Embryology Authority. 2016. *Fertility Treatment in 2014: Trends and Figures*. London: Human Fertilisation and Embryology Authority.

Huxford, J. 2000. "Framing the future: Science fiction frames and the press coverage of cloning." *Continuum* 14 (2): 187–199.

Idiakez, I. A. 2010. "Three decades of reproductive rights: The highs and lows of biomedical innovation." In *Feminist Challenges in the Social Sciences: Gender Studies in the Basque Country*, edited by M. L. Esteban and M. Amurrio, 143–158. Reno, NV: Center for Basque Studies.

Ikemoto, L. C. 2014. "Can human embryonic stem cell research escape its troubled history?" *Hastings Center Report* 44 (6): 7–8.

Inhorn, M. C. 2011. "Globalization and gametes: Reproductive 'tourism,' Islamic bioethics, and Middle Eastern modernity." *Anthropology and Medicine* 18 (1): 87–103.

Inhorn, M. C. 2016. "Cosmopolitan conceptions in global Dubai? The emiratization of IVF and its consequences." *Reproductive Biomedicine and Society Online* 2: 24–31.

Jadva, V., T. Freeman, W. Kramer, and S. Golombok. 2009. "The experiences of adolescents and adults conceived by sperm donation: Comparisons by age of disclosure and family type." *Human Reproduction* 24 (8): 1909–1919.

Jasanoff, S. 2005. *Designs on Nature: Science and Democracy in Europe and the United States*. Princeton, NJ: Princeton University Press.

Jermyn, D. 2008. "Still something else besides a mother? Negotiating celebrity motherhood in Sarah Jessica Parker's star story." *Social Semiotics* 18 (2): 163–176.

Johnson, M. D., A. R. Cooper, E. S. Jungheim, S. E. Lanzendorf, R. R. Odem, and V. S. Ratts. 2013. "Sperm banking for fertility preservation: a 20-year experience." *European Journal of Obstetrics, Gynecology, and Reproductive Biology* 170 (1): 177–182.

Johnston. Josephine, and Miriam Zoll. 2014. "Is freezing your eggs dangerous? A primer." *New Republic*, November 1, 2014. http://www.newrepublic.com/article/120077/dangers-and-realities-egg-freezing.

Jonas, H. 1969. "Philosophical reflections on experimenting with human subjects." *Daedalus* 98: 219–247.

Jørgensen, D. 2013. "Reintroduction and de-extinction." *BioScience* 63 (9): 719–720.

Kannegiesser, H. J. 1988. *Conception in the Test Tube: The IVF Story—How Australia Leads the World*. South Melbourne: Macmillan.

Karpik, L. 2010. *Valuing the Unique: The Economics of Singularities*. Princeton, NJ: Princeton University Press.

Kay, L. E. 2000. *Who Wrote the Book of Life?: A History of the Genetic Code*. Stanford, CA: Stanford University Press.

Keller, E. F. 2000. *The Century of the Gene*. Cambridge, MA: Harvard University Press.

Kiernan, K., H. Land, and J. Lewis. 1998. *Lone Motherhood in Twentieth-Century Britain: From Footnote to Front Page*. Oxford: Oxford University Press.

Klass, D., P. R. Silverman, and S. L. Nickman 1996. *Continuing Bonds: New Understandings of Grief*. Washington, DC: Taylor and Francis.

Kmietowicz, Z. 2015. "UK becomes first country to allow mitochondrial donation." *British Medical Journal* 350: h1103.

Kondapalli, L., F. Hong, and C. Garcia. 2010. "Clinical cases in oncofertility." In *Oncofertility: Ethical, Legal, Social, and Medical Perspectives*, edited by T. Woodruff, L. Zoloth, L. Campo-Engelstein, and S. Rodriguez, 55–67. New York: Springer.

Kristol, W., and E. Cohen, eds. 2002. *The Future Is Now: America Confronts the New Genetics*. New York: Rowman and Littlefield.

Kroløkke, C. 2009. "Click a donor: Viking masculinity on the line." *Journal of Consumer Culture* 9 (1): 7–30.

Kroløkke, C. H. 2014. "West is best: Affective assemblages and Spanish oöcytes." *European Journal of Women's Studies* 21 (1): 57–71.

Kroløkke, C. H., and S. W. Adrian. 2013. "Sperm on ice." *Australian Feminist Studies* 28 (77): 263–278.

Kuleshova, L. L. 2009. "17: Ten years of success in vitrification of human oocytes." *Cryobiology* 59 (3): 374–375.

Kupka, M. S., A. P. Ferraretti, J. de Mouzon, K. Erb, T. D'Hooghe, J. A. Castilla, C. Calhaz-Jorge, C. De Geyter, and V. Goossens. 2014. "Assisted reproductive technology in Europe, 2010: Results generated from European registers by ESHRE." *Human Reproduction* 29 (10): 2099–2113.

Kushnir, V. A., and N. Gleicher 2016. "Fresh versus cryopreserved oocyte donation." *Current Opinion in Endocrinology, Diabetes and Obesity* 23 (6): 451–457.

Landecker, H. 2005. "Living differently in time: Plasticity, temporality and cellular biotechnologies." *Culture Machine* 7 (1). http://www.culturemachine.net/index.php/cm/article/view/26/33.

Latham, K. E. 1999. "Mechanisms and control of embryonic genome activation in mammalian embryos." *International Review of Cytology* 193: 71–124.

Laurence, W. 1936. "Life is generated in scientist's tube: Dr. Pincus of Harvard reports to biologists the first 'semi-ectogenesis' of rabbits." *New York Times*, March 27, 1936.

Lazzaroni-Tealdi, E., D. H. Barad, D. F. Albertini, Y. Yu, V. A. Kushnir, H. Russell, Y.-G. Wu, and N. Gleicher. 2015. "Oocyte scoring enhances embryo-scoring in predicting pregnancy chances with IVF where it counts most." *PLOS ONE* 10 (12): e0143632.

Lee, R. 2009. "New trends in global outsourcing of commercial surrogacy: A call for regulation." *Hastings Women's Law Journal* 20 (2): 275–300.

Leem, S. Y., and J. H. Park. 2008. "Rethinking women and their bodies in the age of biotechnology: Feminist commentaries on the Hwang affair." *East Asian Science, Technology and Society* 2 (1): 9–26.

Leeton, J., and R. Riley. 2013. *Test Tube Revolution: The Early History of IVF.* Clayton, Vic.: Monash University Publishing.

Lemke, T. 2011. "Critique and experience in Foucault." *Theory, Culture and Society* 28 (4): 26–48.

Levine, A. 2010. "Self-regulation, compensation, and the ethical recruitment of oocyte donors." *Hastings Center Report* 40 (2): 25–36.

Lewenhoeck, D. A. 1677. "Observationes D: Anthonii Lewenhoeck, de natis e semine genitali animalculis." *Philosophical Transactions* 12 (133–142): 1040–1046.

Lewis, W. H., and P. W. Gregory. 1929. "Cinematographs of living developing rabbit-eggs." *Science* 69 (1782): 226–229.

Ley, R. E., M. Hamady, C. Lozupone, P. Turnbaugh, R. R. Ramey, J. S. Bircher, M. L. Schlegel, T. A. Tucker, M. D. Schrenzel, R. Knight, and J. I. Gordon. 2008. "Evolution of mammals and their gut microbes." *Science* 320 (5883): 1647–1651.

Lord, J., L. Shaw, F. Dobbs, and U. Acharya. 2001. "A time for change and a time for equality—Infertility services and the NHS." *Human Fertility* 4 (4): 256–260.

Lu, L., B. Lv, K. Huang, Z. Xue, X. Zhu, and G. Fan. 2016. "Recent advances in preimplantation genetic diagnosis and screening." *Journal of Assisted Reproduction and Genetics* 33 (9): 1129–1134.

Lucci, P., and B. Harrison. 2011. *The Knowledge Economy: Reviewing the Make-up of the Knowledge Economy in London.* London: Future of London.

Lutz, H. 2008. *Migration and Domestic Work: A European Perspective on a Global Theme.* Aldershot: Ashgate.

Macaldowie, A., E. Lee, and G. Chambers. 2015. *Assisted Reproductive Technology in Australia and New Zealand 2013.* Sydney: National Perinatal Epidemiology and Statistics Unit, University of New South Wales.

Macaldowie, A., Y. A. Wang, A. A. Chughtai, and G. M. Chambers. 2014. *Assisted Reproductive Technology in Australia and New Zealand 2012.* Sydney: National Perinatal Epidemiology and Statistics Unit, University of New South Wales.

Mackenzie, A. 2013. "Realizing the promise of biotechnology: Infrastructural-icons in synthetic biology." *Futures* 48:5–12.

Mahon, E. 2014. "Assisted reproductive technology—IVF treatment in Ireland: A study of couples with successful outcomes." *Human Fertility* 17 (3): 165–169.

Mamo, L. 2007. *Queering Reproduction: Achieving Pregnancy in the Age of Technoscience*. Durham, NC: Duke University Press.

Mamode, N., A. Lennerling, F. Citterio, E. Massey, K. Van Assche, S. Sterckx, M. Frunza, H. Jung, A. Pascalev, W. Zuidema, R. Johnson, C. Loven, W. Weimar, and F. Dor. 2013. "Anonymity and live-donor transplantation: An ELPAT view." *Transplantation* 95 (4): 536–541.

Margulis, L., and D. Sagan. 1986. *Origins of Sex: Three Billion Years of Genetic Recombination*. New Haven, CT: Yale University Press.

Margulis, L., and D. Sagan. 1997. *Slanted Truths: Essays on Gaia, Symbiosis, and Evolution*. New York: Copernicus.

Martin, E. 1991. "The egg and the sperm: How science has constructed a romance based on stereotypical male-female roles." *Signs* 16:485–501.

Mason, C., and P. Dunnill. 2008. "A brief definition of regenerative medicine." Editorial. *Regenerative Medicine* 3 (1): 1–5.

Melton, Douglas A. 2014. "'Stemness': Definitions, criteria, and standards." In *Essentials of Stem Cell Biology*, edited by R. Lanza and A. Atala, 7–17. Boston: Academic Press.

Miller, T. 2007. *Making Babies: Personal IVF Stories*. Carlton North, Vic.: Scribe.

Mitalipov, S., and D. Wolf. 2009. "Totipotency, pluripotency and nuclear reprogramming." In *Engineering of Stem Cells*, edited by U. Martin, 185–199. Berlin: Springer.

Mohapatra, S. 2014. "Using egg freezing to extend the biological clock: Fertility insurance or false hope?" *Harvard Law and Policy Review* 8:381–412.

Moore, N. 1970. "Preliminary studies on in vitro culture of fertilized sheep ova." *Australian Journal of Biological Science* 23:721–724.

Morgan, L. M. 2009. *Icons of Life: A Cultural History of Human Embryos*. Berkeley: University of California Press.

Mullen, S. F. 2007. "Advances in the Fundamental Cryobiology of Mammalian Oocytes." PhD diss., University of Missouri, Columbia.

Mullen, S. F. 2011. "The evolution of methods to cryopreserve human oocytes." *Cryobiology* 63 (3): 308.

Murphy, D. A. 2013. "The desire for parenthood: Gay men choosing to become parents through surrogacy." *Journal of Family Issues* 34 (8): 1104–1124.

Murphy, M. 2012. *Seizing the Means of Reproduction: Entanglements of Feminism, Health, and Technoscience*. Durham, NC: Duke University Press.

Murray, J. D., and E. A. Maga. 2016. "Genetically engineered livestock for agriculture: A generation after the first transgenic animal research conference." *Transgenic Research* 25 (3): 321–327.

Nahman, M. R. 2013. *Extractions: An Ethnography of Reproductive Tourism*. Basingstoke: Palgrave Macmillan.

National Center for Chronic Disease Prevention and Health Promotion. 2014. *2012 Assisted Reproductive Technology: Fertility Clinic Success Rates Report*. Atlanta, GA: Centers for Disease Control and Prevention, Division of Reproductive Health.

National Health Service. 2013. "IVF." *NHS Choices*, August 1, 2013. http://www .nhs.uk/conditions/IVF/Pages/Introduction.aspx.

Neimanis, A. 2014. "Speculative reproduction: Biotechnologies and ecologies in thick time." *philoSOPHIA: Journal of Continental Feminist Philosophy* 4 (1): 108–128.

Nisker, J., F. Baylis, I. Karpin, C. McLeod, and R. Mykitiuk. 2010. *The 'Healthy' Embryo: Social, Biomedical, Legal and Philosophical Perspectives*. Cambridge: Cambridge University Press.

Noggle, S., H.-L. Fung, A. Gore, H. Martinez, K. C. Satriani, R. Prosser, K. Oum, D. Paull, S. Druckenmiller, M. Freeby, E. Greenberg, K. Zhang, R. Goland, M. V. Sauer, R. L. Leibel, and D. Egli. 2011. "Human oocytes reprogram somatic cells to a pluripotent state." *Nature* 478 (7367): 70–75.

NSW Ministry of Health. 2013. *NSW Health Framework for Women's Health 2013*. Sydney: NSW Health.

Nuffield Council on Bioethics. 2012. *Novel Techniques for the Prevention of Mitochondrial DNA Disorders: An Ethical Review*. London: Nuffield Council on Bioethics.

NYSTEM Strategic Planning Coordinating Committee. 2015. *A Report of the Empire State Stem Cell Board 2015*. Albany: New York State Stem Cell Science (NYSTEM) Program.

OECD. 2006. *The Bioeconomy to 2030: Designing A Policy Agenda*. Paris: OECD.

Oktay, K., A. P. Cil, and H. Bang. 2006. "Efficiency of oocyte cryopreservation: A meta-analysis." *Fertility and Sterility* 86 (1): 70–80.

Oyama, S. 2000. *The Ontogeny of Information: Developmental Systems and Evolution*. Durham, NC: Duke University Press.

Parker, G., R. Baker, and V. Smith. 1972. "The origin and evolution of gamete dimorphism and the male-female phenomenon." *Journal of Theoretical Biology* 36:529–553.

Pennings, G., J. de Mouzon, F. Shenfield, A. P. Ferraretti, T. Mardesic, A. Ruiz, and V. Goossens. 2014. "Socio-demographic and fertility-related characteristics and motivations of oocyte donors in eleven European countries." *Human Reproduction* 29 (5): 1076–1089.

Pincus, G. 1936. *The Eggs of Mammals*. New York: Macmillan.

Polge, C., A. Smith, and A. Parkes. 1949. "Revival of spermatozoa after vitrification and dehydration at low temperatures." *Nature* 164 (4172): 666.

Public Health Association of Australia. 2013. *Public Health Association of Australia: Policy-at-a-Glance–Preconception Health and Fertility Policy*. Curtin, ACT: PHAA.

Quaas, A. M., A. Melamed, K. Chung, K. A. Bendikson, and R. J. Paulson. 2013. "Egg banking in the United States: current status of commercially available cryopreserved oocytes." *Fertility and Sterility* 99 (3): 827–831.

Race, K. 2014. "Speculative pragmatism and intimate arrangements: Online hook-up devices in gay life." *Culture, Health and Sexuality* 17 (4): 496–511.

Radin, J. 2012. "Life on ice: Frozen blood and human biological variation in a genomic age, 1950–2010." PhD diss., University of Pennsylvania.

Radin, J. 2013. "Latent life: Concepts and practices of human tissue preservation in the International Biological Program." *Social Studies of Science* 43 (4): 484–508.

Radin, J., and E. Kowal, eds. 2017a. *Cryopolitics: Frozen Life in a Melting World.* Cambridge, MA: MIT Press.

Radin, J., and E. Kowal. 2017b. "Introduction: The politics of low temperature." *Cryopolitics: Frozen Life in a Melting World*, edited by J. Radin and E. Kowal, 3–26. Cambridge, MA: MIT Press.

Rall, W. F., and G. M. Fahy. 1985. "Ice-free cryopreservation of mouse embryos at −196°C by vitrification." *Nature* 313 (6003): 573–575.

Rapp, R. 1987. "Moral pioneers: Women, men and fetuses on a frontier of reproductive technology." *Women Health* 13 (1/2): 101–116.

Rienzi, L., G. Vajta, and F. Ubaldi. 2011. "Predictive value of oocyte morphology in human IVF: A systematic review of the literature." *Human Reproduction Update* 17 (1): 34–45.

Roberts, E. 2010. "Egg traffic in Ecuador in the context of Latin American reproductive policy." In *Unraveling the Fertility Industry: Challenges and Strategies for Movement Building*, 80–82. New Delhi: SAMA.

Roberts, E. 2012. *God's Laboratory: Assisted Reproduction in the Andes.* Berkeley: University of California Press.

Roemer, I., W. Reik, W. Dean, and J. Klose. 1997. "Epigenetic inheritance in the mouse." *Current Biology* 7 (4): 277–280.

Rose, N., and C. Novas. 2004. "Biological citizenship." In *Global Assemblages: Technology, Politics, and Ethics as Anthropological Problems*, edited by A. Ong and S. J. Collier, 439–463. Oxford: Blackwell.

Roxland, B. E. 2012. "New York State's landmark policies on oversight and compensation for egg donation to stem cell research." *Regenerative Medicine* 7 (3): 397–408.

Ryan, K., V. Team, and J. Alexander. 2013. "Expressionists of the twenty-first century: The commodification and commercialization of expressed breast milk." *Medical Anthropology* 32 (5): 467–486.

Sample, I., and D. Macleod. 2005. "Cloning plan poses new ethical dilemma: Scientist courts controversy with call for women to donate eggs." *Guardian* (Manchester), July 26, 2005.

Sarnat, H. B., and M. G. Netsky. 2002. "When does a ganglion become a brain? Evolutionary origin of the central nervous system." *Seminars in Pediatric Neurology* 9 (4): 240–253.

Schover, L. R. 2014. "Cross-border surrogacy: The case of Baby Gammy highlights the need for global agreement on protections for all parties." *Fertility and Sterility* 102 (5): 1258–1259.

Scott, J. W. 1992. "The evidence of experience." In *Feminists Theorise the Political*, edited by J. W. Scott and J. Butler, 22–40. New York: Routledge.

Shane, S. 2012. "I've frozen my eggs while I find Mr Right." *Grazia Daily UK*, December 4, 57–58.

Shapiro, B. 2015. *How to Clone a Mammoth: The Science of De-Extinction*. Princeton, NJ: Princeton University Press.

Sheikh, S. 2013. *Medical Frontiers: Debating Mitochondria Replacement: Patient Focus Group Report to* HFEA. London: Office of Public Management.

Shenfield, F., J. de Mouzon, G. Pennings, A. P. Ferraretti, A. Nyboe Andersen, G. de Wert, and V. Goossens. 2010. "Cross border reproductive care in six European countries." *Human Reproduction* 25 (6): 1361–1368.

Shkedi-Rafid, S., and Y. Hashiloni-Dolev. 2011. "Egg freezing for age-related fertility decline: preventive medicine or a further medicalization of reproduction? Analyzing the new Israeli policy." *Fertility and Sterility* 96 (2): 291–294.

Short, R. 2003. "The magic and mystery of the oocyte: *ex ovo omnia*." In *Biology and Pathology of the Oocyte. Role in Fertility and Reproductive Medicine*, edited by A. Trounson and R. Gosden, 3–10. Cambridge: Cambridge University Press.

Shuster, A. 1969. "Human egg fertilized in test tube by Britons." *New York Times*, February 15, 1969.

Skeggs, B. 2004. *Class, Self, Culture*. London: Routledge.

Slabbert, M. N., and M. S. Pepper. 2015. "A global comparative overview of the legal regulation of stem cell research and therapy: Lessons for South Africa." *South African Journal of Bioethics and Law* 8 (2 Suppl 1): 12–22.

Smith, G. D., P. C. Serafini, J. Fioravanti, I. Yadid, M. Coslovsky, P. Hassun, J. R. Alegretti, and E. L. Motta. 2010. "Prospective randomized comparison of human oocyte cryopreservation with slow-rate freezing or vitrification." *Fertility and Sterility* 94 (6): 2088–2095.

Stewart, J. B., and P. F. Chinnery. 2015. "The dynamics of mitochondrial DNA heteroplasmy: Implications for human health and disease." *Nature Review Genetics* 16 (9): 530–542.

Storper, M., and A. J. Scott. 2009. "Rethinking human capital, creativity and urban growth." *Journal of Economic Geography* 9 (2): 147–167.

Stuart-Smith, S. J., J. A. Smith, and E. J. Scott. 2012. "To know or not to know? Dilemmas for women receiving unknown oocyte donation." *Human Reproduction* 27 (7): 2067–2075.

Syrett, S., and L. Sepulveda. 2012. "Urban governance and economic development in the diverse city." *European Urban and Regional Studies* 19 (3): 238–253.

Tachibana, M., P. Amato, M. Sparman, N. M. Gutierrez, R. Tippner-Hedges, H. Ma, E. Kang, A. Fulati, H. S. Lee, H. Sritanaudomchai, K. Masterson, J. Larson, D. Eaton, K. Sadler-Fredd, D. Battaglia, D. Lee, D. Wu, J. Jensen, P. Patton, S. Gokhale, R. L. Stouffer, D. Wolf, and S. Mitalipov. 2013. "Human embryonic stem cells derived by somatic cell nuclear transfer." *Cell* 153 (6): 1228–1238.

Tadros, W., and H. D. Lipshitz. 2009. "The maternal-to-zygotic transition: A play in two acts." *Development* 136 (18): 3033–3042.

Terman, S. 2008. "Marketing motherhood: Rights and responsibilities of egg donors in assisted reproductive technology agreements." *Northwestern Journal of Law and Social Policy* 3 (1): 167–184.

Thompson, C. 2005. *Making Parents: The Ontological Choreography of Reproductive Technologies.* Cambridge, MA: MIT Press.

Thompson, C. 2007. "Why we should, in fact, pay for egg donation." *Regenerative Medicine* 2 (2): 203–209.

Thompson, C. 2013. *Good Science: The Ethical Choreography of Stem Cell Research.* Cambridge, MA: MIT Press.

Throsby, K. 2002. "'Vials, ampoules and a bucketful of syringes': The experience of the self-administration of hormonal drugs in IVF." *Feminist Review* 72 (1): 62–77.

Throsby, K. 2004. *When IVF Fails: Feminism, Infertility, and the Negotiation of Normality.* Basingstoke: Palgrave Macmillan.

Titmuss, R. M. (1970) 1997. *The Gift Relationship: From Human Blood to Social Policy.* London: LSE Books.

Tober, D. M. 2001. "Semen as gift, semen as goods: Reproductive workers and the market in altruism." *Body and Society* 7 (2/3): 137–160.

Tonkin, L. 2012. "Haunted by a 'present absence.'" *Studies in the Maternal* 4 (1): 1–17.

Tran, M. 2014. "Kirstie Allsopp tells young women: Ditch university and have a baby by 27." *Guardian* (Manchester), June 2, 2014.

Trounson, A. O. 1974. "Studies on the development of fertilized sheep ova." PhD diss., University of Sydney.

Trounson, A., W. Chamley, J. Kennedy, and R. Tassell. 1974. "Primordial follicle numbers in ovaries and levels of LH and FSH in pituitaries and plasma of lambs selected for and against multiple births." *Australian Journal of Biological Sciences* 27 (3): 293–300.

Trounson, A., and Natalie D. DeWitt. 2013. "Pluripotent stem cells from cloned human embryos: Success at long last." *Cell Stem Cell* 12 (6): 636–638.

Trounson, A., and R. Godsen, eds. 2003. *Biology and Pathology of the Oocyte: Role in Fertility and Reproductive Medicine.* Cambridge: Cambridge University Press.

Trounson, A., J. Leeton, M. Besanko, C. Wood, and A. Conti 1983. "Pregnancy established in an infertile patient after transfer of a donated embryo fertilized in vitro." *British Medical Journal* 286: 835–838.

Trounson, A., and N. Moore. 1972. "Ovulation rate and survival of fertilized ova in Merino ewes selected for and against multiple births." *Crop and Pasture Science* 23 (5): 851–858.

Trounson, A., and N. Moore. 1974. "Attempts to produce identical offspring in the sheep by mechanical division of the ovum." *Australian Journal of Biological Sciences* 27 (5): 505–510.

Tucker, M. J., J. Lim, M. VerMilyea, and M. J. Levy. 2012. "Human oocyte cryopreservation and its expanding utilization in assisted reproductive technology." *U.S. Obstetrics and Gynecology* 7 (1): 40–43.

Twenge, J. 2013. "Is it really too late to have a baby?" *Observer Magazine,* July 14, 24–29.

UNESCO. 1997. *Universal Declaration on the Human Genome and Human Rights.* Paris: UNESCO.

van der Wijst, M. G. P., and M. G. Rots. 2015. "Mitochondrial epigenetics: An overlooked layer of regulation?" *Trends in Genetics* 31 (7): 353–356.

Victorian Assisted Reproductive Treatment Authority. 2012. *Annual Report 2012.* Melbourne: Victorian Assisted Reproductive Treatment Authority.

Victorian Assisted Reproductive Treatment Authority. 2013. *Guidelines for the Import and Export of Donor Gametes and Embryos Produced from Donor Gametes.* Melbourne: Victorian Assisted Reproductive Treatment Authority.

Victorian Assisted Reproductive Treatment Authority. 2014. *Annual Report 2014.* Melbourne: Victorian Assisted Reproductive Treatment Authority.

Waldby, C. 1983. "The political regulation of motherhood in Australia: 1880–1914." Honours diss., University of Sydney.

Waldby, C. 1996. *AIDS and the Body Politic: Biomedicine and Sexual Difference.* London: Routledge.

Waldby, C. 2000. *The Visible Human Project: Informatic Bodies and Posthuman Medicine.* London: Routledge.

Waldby, C. 2002. "Biomedicine, tissue transfer and intercorporeality." *Feminist Theory* 3 (3): 235–250.

Waldby, C. 2006. "Umbilical cord blood: From social gift to venture capital." *BioSocieties* 1 (1): 55–70.

Waldby, Catherine. 2015a "'Banking time': Egg freezing, internet dating and the negotiation of future fertility." *Culture, Health and Sexuality: An International Journal for Research, Intervention and Care* 17 (4): 470–482.

Waldby, Catherine. 2015b "The oocyte market and social egg freezing: From scarcity to singularity." *Journal of Cultural Economy* 8 (3): 275–291.

Waldby, C., and K. Carroll. 2012. "Egg donation for stem cell research: Ideas of surplus and deficit in Australian IVF patients' and reproductive donors' accounts." *Sociology of Health and Illness* 34 (4): 513–528.

Waldby, C., and M. Cooper. 2008. "The biopolitics of reproduction: Post-Fordist biotechnology and women's clinical labour." In "The Two Cultures," special issue, *Australian Feminist Studies* 23 (55): 57–73.

Waldby, C., and M. Cooper. 2010. "From reproductive work to regenerative labour: The female body and the stem cell industries." *Feminist Theory* 11 (1): 3–22.

Waldby, C., I. Kerridge, M. Boulos, and K. Carroll. 2013. "From altruism to monetisation: Australian women's ideas about money, ethics and research eggs." *Social Science and Medicine* 94: 34–42.

Waldby, C., I. Kerridge, and L. Skene. 2012. "Multidisciplinary perspectives on the donation of stem cells and reproductive tissue." *Journal of Bioethical Inquiry* 9 (1): 15–17.

Waldby, C., and R. Mitchell. 2006. *Tissue Economies: Blood, Organs and Cell Lines in Late Capitalism.* Durham, NC: Duke University Press.

Waldby, C., M. Rosengarten, C. Treloar, and S. Fraser. 2004. "Blood and bioidentity: Ideas about self, boundaries and risk among blood donors and people living with hepatitis C." *Social Science and Medicine* 59 (7): 1461–1471.

Webster, A. 2011. *Regenerative Medicine in Europe: Emerging Needs and Challenges in a Global Context: Project Final Report Brussels European Commission.* Luxembourg: EU Publications.

Weismann, A. 1892. *The Germ Plasm: A Theory of Heredity.* New York: Scribner.

White House. 2012. *National Bioeconomy Blueprint.* Washington, DC: White House.

Whittaker, A. 2016. "From 'Mung Ming' to 'Baby Gammy': A local history of assisted reproduction in Thailand." *Reproductive Biomedicine and Society Online* 2: 71–78.

Whittaker, A., and A. Speier. 2010. "Cycling overseas: Care, commodification, and stratification in cross-border reproductive travel." *Medical Anthropology: Cross-Cultural Studies in Health and Illness* 29 (4): 363–383.

Williams, R. 1977. *Marxism and Literature.* Oxford: Oxford University Press.

Williams, R. 1983. *Keywords: A Vocabulary of Culture and Society*. London: Fontana.

Wilmot, S. 2007a. "Between the farm and the clinic: Agriculture and reproductive technology in the twentieth century." *Studies in History and Philosophy of Science Part C: Studies in History and Philosophy of Biological and Biomedical Sciences* 38 (2): 303–315.

Wilmot, S. 2007b. "From 'public service' to artificial insemination: Animal breeding science and reproductive research in early twentieth-century Britain." *Studies in History and Philosophy of Science Part C: Studies in History and Philosophy of Biological and Biomedical Sciences* 38 (2): 411–441.

Wilmut, I., A. E. Schnieke, J. McWhir, A. J. Kind, and K. H. Campbell. 1997. "Viable offspring derived from fetal and adult mammalian cells." *Nature* 385 (6619): 810–813.

Woods, R. J. H. 2017. Nature and the refrigerating machine: The politics and production of cold in the nineteenth century." In *Cryopolitics: Frozen Life in a Melting World*, edited by J. Radin and E. Kowal, 89–116. Cambridge, MA: MIT Press.

Yamada, M., B. Johannesson, I. Sagi, L. C. Burnett, D. H. Kort, R. W. Prosser, D. Paull, M. W. Nestor, M. Freeby, E. Greenberg, R. S. Goland, R. L. Leibel, S. L. Solomon, N. Benvenisty, M. V. Sauer, and D. Egli. 2014. "Human oocytes reprogram adult somatic nuclei of a type 1 diabetic to diploid pluripotent stem cells." *Nature* 510 (7506): 533–536.

Zamostny, K. P., K. M. O'Brien, A. L. Baden, and M. O. L. Wiley. 2003. "The practice of adoption: History, trends, and social context." *Counseling Psychologist* 31 (6): 651–678.

Zelizer, V. A. R. 1994. *Pricing the Priceless Child: The Changing Social Value of Children*. Princeton, NJ: Princeton University Press.

Zimmerman, M. K., J. S. Litt, and C. E. Bose. 2006. *Global Dimensions of Gender and Carework*. Stanford, CA: Stanford Social Sciences.

Index

....

eggs. *See* oocytes; zygotes

egg sharing, 11, 89, 94–95, 105, 176–77

Eggs of Mammals, The (Pincus), 48

Egli Laboratory, 178

Elder, Kay, 58–61

EMA (European Medicines Agency), 135

embryogenesis, 29, 32, 35–38, 48–49, 86, 115

embryology, 44–45, 48. *See also* experiment and experience; IVF

embryos: disposal of unused, 78–79, 127, 207n3 (chap. 3); legal protection for, 91; multiple transfers of, 126–27; regulations regarding, 91–92, 207n4 (chap. 4) (*see also under* Australia; United Kingdom). *See also* cryopreservation of oocytes/tissues

empathic intersubjectivity, 13

Empire State Stem Cell Board, 177

empirical experimentation. *See* experiment and experience

Enlightenment science, 44

ESHRE (European Society for Human Reproduction and Embryology), 123

ethics of care, 195

ethics of oocyte regulation, 22, 191–98

eukaryotes, 29–30

European Medicines Agency (EMA), 135

European Society for Human Reproduction and Embryology (ESHRE), 123

European Union (EU): oocyte market in, 90, 98–101; oocyte procurement/management in, 104; regulations regarding tissue donation, 11, 98–99, 138

EU Tissue and Cells Directive, 98–99, 104

evolutionary biology, 25–26, 30–31

experience, generally, 13–14

experiment and experience, 41–63; artificial insemination (AI), 47,

53–54; desire for children and medicalization of infertility, 41–42, 50–53; embryo transfer, 45–46, 48; and informed consent, 61; in vivo oocytes and reproductive biology, 44–50; IVF, history of, 18–19, 47–49, 53–62; overview of, 18–19, 41–44, 62–63; test tube women, 50, 56–62, 64; Williams on, 15

extinction reversal via cloning, 162

family planning organizations, 52

FDA (U.S. Food and Drug Administration), 135

feminists: on gendered qualities of gametes, 27–28, 35; on the limits of femininity and reproduction, 43–44; self-help advocated by, 52–53; on stem cell research, 168; on women's willingness to risk new reproductive technologies, 15

fertility: celebration of late motherhood, 11; fertile time, 17; fertility cliff, 11, 65, 149–50; medicalization of infertility, 41–42, 50–53

fertility and deep time, 23–40; anisogamy, 18, 31–33; biological clock, 11, 23–24, 33–34, 126; and Dolly the sheep, 9, 25, 38–39, 206n2 (chap. 1); and evolutionary biology, 25–26, 30–31; generational continuity of gametes, 18; and generational time, 26–27; mammalian sex, 27–31; overview of, 18, 23–27; temporalities, fertile, 23, 39–40; and thick time, 24–25; totipotency, 18, 25, 34–39

Fertility is Ageist, 65

form/matter distinction, 35

Foucault, Michel, 14

Fowler, Ruth, 53–54

France, 20

Franklin, Sarah, 35, 38, 45, 68, 161–62

freezing eggs/embryos. *See* cryopreservation of oocytes/tissues; egg banking, personal; egg banks, corporate

FSH (follicle-stimulating hormone), 70–72, 154–55

Gamete and Embryo Donation Ref: 0001 (United Kingdom), 208n5

gametes, 7–8; active sperm vs. passive egg, 27–28; and cytobiology, 28; dimorphism of, 31–32; and generational time, 158; mammalian sex, 27–31. *See also* oocytes; sperm; zygotes

Gates, Alan, 53–54

Gaudillière, Jean-Paul, 46–47

gene centrism, 34–35, 38

generational time: and cloning, 164; communicated via oocytes, 7–8, 26–27; definition of, 8, 26; and egg banking, 21–22, 146–47, 157–59; and egg donor matching, 117; women's agency in, 27

genomes, 25, 29–30, 36–37, 187, 189

Germany, 91–92, 207n4 (chap. 4)

germ line modification, ban on, 183–84

Greece, 101–2

Gregory, Paul, 48

Grosz, Elizabeth, 30–31

Haeckel, Ernst, 45

Haimes, Erica, 75, 185–86

Haldane, J. B. S., 57; *Daedalus, or, Science and the Future*, 206n4

Harvey, William: *De Generatione Animalum*, 44

Health Canada, 135

Heape, Walter, 45–46, 48

HeLa controversy, 175

Herbert Laboratory, 177

HFEA (Human Fertilisation and Embryology Authority), 138–39, 147, 165–66, 186, 188, 193–94, 207n2 (chap. 4)

HFE Act (Human Fertilisation and Embryology Act; United Kingdom, 1990, 2008), 139, 180, 183–84, 207nn1–2 (chap. 4), 208n5

His, Wilhelm, 45

HPG (human pituitary gonadotrophin), 62

human cloning, 80, 164–66, 208n5. *See also* cloning, mammalian

Human Fertilisation and Embryology Act. *See* HFE Act

Human Fertilisation and Embryology Authority. *See* HFEA

human pituitary gonadotrophin (HPG), 62

Huntington chorea, 182

husbandry, industrial, 46–47, 62

Huxley, Aldous: *Brave New World*, 57, 206n4

Hwang (Woo Suk) scandal (2005), 11, 90, 167–68, 175, 206n5

ICSI (intracytoplasmic sperm injection), 66–67, 74–75, 207n2 (chap. 3)

immortalized cells, 2, 175

immune system, 1–2

infertility. *See* fertility; fertility and deep time

informed consent, 61, 175, 198

Inovulation (Beaty), 48

Institute of Medicine, 183

internet dating, 152

intracytoplasmic sperm injection (ICSI), 66–67, 74–75, 207n2 (chap. 3)

in vitro fertilization. *See* IVF

iPSCs (induced pluripotent stem cells), 163, 179

Iranian oocyte market, 90

Ireland, 80

ISCO Oceanside, 176

Our Bodies, Ourselves, 52
ovarian reserve, 31–33, 154–57
Oviedo Convention, 98–99, 208n5
Oyama, Susan, 34

Pennings, Guido, 81, 100–101
PGD (preimplantation genetic diagnosis), 66–67, 180, 182
Pill, the, 19, 51
Pincus, Gregory, 57; *The Eggs of Mammals*, 48
Polge, Christopher, 121
population control, 52
potential, degrees of, 37–38. *See also* totipotency
preimplantation genetic diagnosis (PGD), 66–67, 180, 182
Pro Choice Alliance for Responsible Research, 176
Prohibition of Human Cloning and the Regulation of Human Embryo Research Amendment Act (Australia, 2006), 80, 166
Prohibition of Human Cloning for Reproduction Act (Australia, 2002), 208n5
Purdy, Jean, 53, 56–59

queer family formation, 20, 112

rainbow adoption/family, 20, 112, 118
Reed, Candice, 56, 61
regenerative medicine, 40
Renard, J.-P., 36–37
Reproductive Health and Research Bill (California, 2006), 176
Reproductive Technology Accreditation Committee (RTAC), 140–41
research: experience and methodology, 12–17, 206n6; fieldwork and data, 9–11, 205n4. *See also* cloning, therapeutic; SCNT
Roberts, Elizabeth, 111–12, 118

Royal Society of London, 183
RTAC (Reproductive Technology Accreditation Committee), 140–41

Sagan, Dorian, 28–32, 35–36
San Francisco, 11, 125
Schultz, Susanne, 10, 176–77
SCNT (somatic cell nuclear transfer):
Dolly the sheep produced via, 38–39, 206n2 (chap. 1); funding for, 11; human SCNT lines established, 178; Hwang scandal involving, 11, 90, 167–68, 175, 206n5; legislation surrounding, 165, 208n5; and oocyte capacities, 38; technique of, 38–39; time, labor, and payment issues in egg donation, 169–79; use in therapeutic cloning, 9, 164–69
Scott, Joan, 13–14
self-help movement, 52–53
sex, mammalian, 27–31
sexuality and household formation, 152–54, 194
Sidebotham, Mary, 81
singularity value, 146
social egg freezing. *See* egg banking, personal
somatic cell nuclear transfer. *See* SCNT
South African oocyte market, 90, 102–4
South Korea, 90, 167–68. *See also* Hwang scandal
Spain, 80, 92, 99, 101, 104–6, 139, 142, 177
sperm: capacitation of, 49; donation of, 114–15; motility of, 31–32; production of, 32; size of, vs. oocytes, 31–32, 35, 206n1 (chap. 1); sperm banks, 119–20, 135; tails of, 30
Stemagen, 176–77
stem cells, 8–9, 32, 37–38, 40, 66, 163, 165–67. *See also* SCNT
Steptoe, Patrick, 53–54, 56–61